THE PUBLIC HEALTH OBSERVATORY HANDBOOK OF HEALTH INEQUALITIES MEASUREMENT

Roy Carr-Hill, Paul Chalmers-Dixon

Centre for Health Economics, University of York

Edited by Jennifer Lin
Visiting Research Fellow at the South East Public Health Observatory

2005

South East Public Health Observatory
4150 Chancellor Court
Oxford Business Park South
Oxford OX4 2GX
www.sepho.org.uk

ISBN: 0-9542971-2-1

Table of Contents

LIST OF TABLES

Preface

Tackling health inequalities must be a central plank of public policy for any government, so I was honoured to be asked to undertake the review of health inequalities for the Labour Government in 1998. I hope that the report from the review, "The Independent Enquiry into Inequalities in Health", has helped to shape the policy direction, and influence the targeting and delivery of services, in tackling inequalities.

We have moved a long way in our commitment to tackle health inequalities since then. The evidence base about "what works" is still fairly weak, but there is now a commitment to address this. Resources are going into research and development to advance our knowledge and understanding of what works. In parallel with that we need to be able to measure inequalities, in order to plan, set targets, monitor and evaluate. I recommended in my report the need to establish mechanisms to monitor inequalities in health and to evaluate the effectiveness of measures taken to reduce them.

This book is therefore a welcome contribution to the resources available to people working to reduce inequalities in health in their communities. I commend it to anyone involved in addressing health inequalities. The measurement of inequalities is a complicated and convoluted science, but this book brings together much of that science in a rigorous but accessible way. It is a rich source of information and will contribute to advancing our knowledge and practice, with the ultimate aim to reduce inequalities and to make this country a more equitable society.

Sir Donald Acheson

Foreword

The White Paper "Saving Lives: Our Healthier Nation" (Department of Health, 1999) proposed the establishment of Public Health Observatories (PHOs), one in each NHS region of the country, to strengthen the availability and use of information about health at local level. The Public Health Observatories were launched in 2000 by Yvette Cooper, Parliamentary Under Secretary of State for Public Health, and Liam Donaldson, Chief Medical Officer. The White Paper proposed that the role of Public Health Observatories would be to support local bodies by:

- Monitoring health and disease trends and highlighting areas for action.
- Identifying gaps in health information.
- Advising on methods for health impact assessments.
- Drawing together information from different sources in new ways to improve health.
- Carrying out projects to highlight particular health issues.
- Evaluating progress made by local agencies in improving health and reducing inequality.
- Looking ahead to give early warning of future public health problems.

Observatories are now well established and well recognised in their role of supporting public health in England. As part of this, Observatories are making a major contribution in the area of measuring and monitoring inequalities in health. For example:

- We have developed a local basket of indicators for use by local authorities and primary care trusts, to help them identify needs and to monitor and evaluate local public health programmes.
- We have developed the Health Poverty Index (HPI), an index announced in the NHS Plan, that combines data about each population's health status, access to health services, uptake of preventive services and the opportunities to pursue and maintain good health.
- We have been commissioned by the Chief Medical Officer to produce a series of reports presenting indicators of public health for the English Regions. The first of these reports was published in January 2004.

In addition to providing our stakeholders with local intelligence, they have asked us to provide them with methodological advice and support. In the South East Region, people requested the South East Public Health Observatory to develop a resource to assist them with the methodological issues in measuring health inequalities. The South East Public Health

Observatory commissioned this work from Roy Carr-Hill and Paul Dixon, at the University of York. This book is the outcome of that request.

We hope that this book will be useful for all those involved in measuring health inequalities for both policy and practice. The book, commissioned by the English Public Health Observatories, inevitability has an English focus, but we believe it will be of use to people from other parts of the United Kingdom and to people in other countries.

This is the first version of this book. The on-line format allows for frequent updating. Thus, please let us have all your comments and feedback so that we can continually improve it. In addition, a published edition will be available in the near future.

Alison Hill
Programme Director,
South East Public Health Observatory

Michael Goldacre
Scientific Director,
South East Public Health Observatory

John Wilkinson
Chairman,
Association of Public Health Observatories

Acknowledgements

This work was commissioned by the South East Public Health Observatory (SEPHO). We are very grateful to the support we have had from people at SEPHO. We would also like to thank all the readers, recruited by SEPHO to assess an early draft for its relevance to their needs. We hope that we have taken account of many of their comments and are sure the work has benefited as a result. Several people at York University have provided invaluable support to this project, including Elizabeth Currie, Michelle Ellwood, and Rachel Potts.

This handbook was ably edited by Jennifer Lin, visiting Research Fellow at the South East Public Health Observatory.

Feedback

Although theories on the nature and origins of inequality emerge and evolve quite slowly, this is an area in which results and data sources are continually changing and expanding. We have tried to present an overview of those national data sources that provide consistent information on local areas, but are aware that our information may be incomplete and that we have not had the resources to investigate the many local and regional sources. We are also aware of the volatility of web addresses, thus in this version of the handbook have concentrated on the names of the sources or providers, rather than providing web addresses that may soon be outdated.
Any suggestions of sources or comments in the text are encouraged. The simplest way of providing feedback, for future versions, is through the 'interactive pdf' on the SEPHO website (www.sepho.org.uk/Rch_handbook/.)

SECTION 1

INTRODUCTION

The existence and persistence of inequalities in health has been a matter of public record and commentary in the U.K. for a very long time. In fact, the Registrar General's Social Class Classification was designed for use with the 1911 Census, in order to help search for an explanation for differences in fertility and mortality between the industrial proletariat and the wealthier classes [1].

In 1980, discussion on the issue was re-ignited by the partial suppression by the Conservative Government of the report on inequalities in health commissioned under the previous Labour Government (the Black Report) 'Inequalities in Health' [2]. Scholars in other European countries quickly documented similar kinds of disparities between the health status of groups defined by a variety of socio-economic categorisations, and by 1987, the European Region of the World Health Organisation (WHO) adopted the reduction of 25% in health inequalities as the first target of its 'Health for All' by the Year 2000 programme.

Most of the topics addressed in this manual have already been the subject of extensive review. The measurement of inequality in general has been comprehensively reviewed by Atkinson [3], while Bowling [4] and Wilkin et al. [5] have reviewed the measures for measuring health in both clinical and community settings. Equally, various measures of deprivation have been reviewed by Morris and Carstairs [6]; and the problems of measuring socio-economic inequalities in health have been reviewed by Kunst and Mackenbach, Valkonen and Wagstaff [7–9].

All these works have provided excellent starting points, although they have not always been clear on the criteria they use to include and evaluate measures, and the suitability of these criteria for the tasks initially proposed.[1]

---

[1] For example, the analysis by Morris and Carstairs [6] focussed on the comparative performance of different measures of deprivation with the same criterion (whether use of medical care, or morbidity, or mortality), whilst from another perspective, it is the comparative performance of any given deprivation measure *across* criteria which is of interest.

However, none of them bring together, in an easily accessible form, all the relevant issues.

1.1 Inequality and its Measurement

The existence of substantial and persisting inequalities in health and particularly in death is rarely disputed, but there have been contentious arguments over:

- The extent of these inequalities and whether they are increasing or decreasing.
- The causes of the inequalities observed.
- Appropriate methods of measurement and monitoring them.
- What can be done about them.

Existing research in the U.K.

Whilst there is a substantial corpus of research in the U.K. in this area, this has not always served to clarify these questions. In many cases, there has been a confusion in methods of measurement with analysis of the extent of inequalities, or of their causes.

The Health for All 2000 WHO initiative

In contrast, the WHO European Region, faced with a similar task for their Regional Observatories, commissioned a review of methods which could be used by countries in monitoring their progress towards the Health for All by the Year 2000 target [7]. Their's is a clear summary of many of the issues covered in this handbook. Kunst and Mackenbach [7] focussed on the technical properties of the methods of measurement, using concrete analyses to illustrate different methods, but did not use the findings of the analysis as a reason for excluding some methods and privileging others. However, the review was limited to classic socio-economic status measures (occupation, education and income) and to measures of mortality and generalised measures of health. Socio-economic status is an important group classifier but so are, for example, gender and location, amongst others.

1.2 This Handbook

This handbook aims to provide a more comprehensive collection of material for those concerned to document and understand inequalities in health in their area. This includes people working at all levels in the health care sector.

The handbook focuses on the measurement of inequalities in health (and death); inequalities in access to healthcare or quality of care are not explicitly considered. Nevertheless, the issue of the measurement of inequality is quite general, and much of the methodological material will be useful to those working in other sectors. The intention is to provide a *menu* of possible dimensions of inequality and methods of measuring and monitoring inequalities to which the local researcher can refer.

1.3 Core Issues Addressed by the Handbook

There are two basic issues in the measurement of inequalities in health:

- What is meant by inequality?
- How to measure inequality?

What is meant by inequality

Three concepts are frequently used:

- *Differences* or *variations* in health (or income) between groups.
- *Inequalities* in health(or income).
- *Inequities* or the unfairness of differences.

These issues are discussed in Section 10 of the handbook. In this handbook, the term 'variations' is reserved for purely statistical usage and 'inequalities' is used in its descriptive sense. Although the fairness of the differences in health between groups is not discussed here, the purpose of measuring inequalities is because they point to *likely* inequities.

> Kunst and Mackenbach use the following working definition of health inequalities: "Differences in the prevalence or incidence of health problems between individual people of higher and lower socio-economic status" (1995)

It should be emphasised that although the definition refers to individuals, *the crucial characteristic is their membership of one group rather than another*. Whilst differences between individuals may well be interesting in themselves, they are only meaningful in terms of inequity if those differences are linked to the membership of a group.

How to measure inequality

Most measurement of health inequality involves the use of indicators or indexes to measure health, but it also involves decisions on what groups or areas to compare and what is the most appropriate form of analysis for the question being investigated.

In short, devising a method for measuring inequalities requires answers to six questions:

- What is the comparator, are inequalities to be measured between:
  - Groups or populations of small areas (Section 2).
  - Countries or populations to which different socio-economic classification have been applied (Sections 2 and 10).
  - Similar groups or populations over time (Section 10).
- What type of inequality is of interest:
  - Relative or absolute inequality (Sections 9 and 10).
  - Risk-based versus outcome-based measures (Section 10).
- What is the intended use for the index of inequality:
  - To monitor the impact of policies on specific populations (Sections 10 and 11).
  - To compile league tables (Sections 10 and 11).
- What indicator/marker of inequality to choose:
  - Socio-economic categories (Section 2).
  - A deprivation index (Sections 5 and 6).
  - A single variable or an index (Section 7).
- What indicator of health to choose:
  - Routine health data (Section 3).
  - Data from surveys (Sections 4 and 9).
- What data source to use:
  - Existing data sources (Section 8).
  - Generating your own survey data (Section 9).

The importance of distinguishing between methods and results

When measuring inequalities, it is soon apparent that different methods of constructing indexes and different approaches to analysis can give different results or suggest different causes for inequality. One problem with the debates on the nature and extent of inequalities and the direction of historical trends (Section 11) has been that some researchers have tended to privilege the measures and methods that lead to a pre-determined conclusion. Hence, it is always important to understand the relationship between the methods and the results.

1.4 Structure of This Handbook

This handbook tries to address these issues in a practical manner, with each section covering a different stage in the measurement and interpretation of health inequalities.

It is divided into eleven sections:

1. Introduction.
2. Measuring inequality by social categories.
3. Measuring inequality by health and disease categories (using data from administrative sources).
4. Measuring inequality by health and disease categories (using data from surveys).
5. Measuring deprivation with indexes – introduction and summary.
6. Measuring deprivation with indexes – a selection of indexes.
7. The properties of the tools for measuring inequality: what is an index and how is it tested?
8. Overview of existing data sources, availability and problems.
9. Designing surveys to measure inequality.
10. Inequalities and methods of measurement.
11. Context, history and theories of inequality.

In general, the sections address the following questions.

What groups or areas are thought to be unequal? (Section 2)

An early decision in the investigation of inequalities is to specify the types of groups, such as social classes, income groups, or geographical areas, between which inequalities may exist. Section 2 provides a discussion of various socio-demographic, socio-economic and other classifiers that might be used to document inequalities. Definitional issues are raised in relation to each of the topics, as well as questions of data quality and availability.

In what respects are they unequal? (Sections 3–6)

A second decision relates to the dimension of inequality to be investigated. Sections 3 and 4 present a wide range of measures of health that should be suitable for detecting inequalities. Sections 5 and 6 summarise most of the U.K. deprivation indexes which are used to measure inequality, but also have a role in defining groups or areas for the purposes of investigating other forms of inequality, such as differences in health.

What is an index and how is it tested? (Section 7)

Measures of health and deprivation often take the form of indicators and indexes, formulae that combine different characteristics of a phenomenon in order to provide some overall score or ranking. Section 7 unpacks some of the technical characteristics of indexes and introduces some of the methods used in their development and testing.

Obtaining data on inequalities (Sections 8 and 9)

Most measures of health and deprivation rely on data from surveys or administrative systems, such as NHS hospital admissions, and Department of Health (DH) and Social Security benefit systems. Some measures combine material from both types of sources.

Sections 8 and 9 give general advice on obtaining relevant data. Section 8 gives a brief introduction to designing a survey to collect data on inequality and Section 9 introduces some of the more substantial data sources and archives.

How to measure, represent and interpret inequalities (Section 10)

The instruments that measure the dimensions of inequality will provide scores or rankings, or some other form of metric, but they do not always provide an adequate summary of the extent of inequalities. For this, it may be necessary to use some type of summary measure, such as the Gini coefficient. The chosen measure will be related to the study design, e.g. cross-sectional or longitudinal. The choice will also reflect one's interpretation of the nature and meaning of inequality. Section 10 introduces issues on the representation and interpretation of inequalities, together with some of the commonly used summary measures.

The historical and theoretical context (Section 11)

At almost every stage in the investigation of inequality, decisions about the measures to use, the dimensions to investigate, the type of design to adopt and the type of summary measure to employ are likely to influence the results. This is not a pure science. Choices are informed by inherently biased views on the likely nature, extent, and causes of inequality. Section 11 introduces and compares some of the theories to measuring inequality.

Box 1

Example

The Department of Health Inequalities Programme has established a national target on infant mortality.

"Starting with children under one year, by 2010 to reduce by at least 10 per cent the gap in mortality between manual groups and the population as a whole."

- Issues relevant to the types of measurement that are necessary to monitor progress towards this target, and the nature of the target itself, are discussed at various points in the handbook.
- The classifier used to document inequality is the Registrar General's classification of social class (Sections 2 and 7 address the nature and properties of this classification) including the point, that the Department of Health admits that social class is based on father's occupation, and hence is not available for births registered by the mother only.
- The dimension of inequality is infant mortality (based on 3-year averages). Section 8 details how this is computed, possible alternatives, and where to obtain these data. The measure is the mortality rate, but is restricted to those records for which infant deaths could be linked to a birth record.
- The method of analysis, presentation and interpretation involves comparison of 3-year averages (and in some cases year rates) for two social groupings defined by social class. The logic, purpose and limitations of such a comparison are considered in Sections 10 and 11.

SECTION 2

MEASURING INEQUALITY BY SOCIAL CATEGORIES

2.1 Introduction

This section looks at the different group classifiers or categories that are usually employed in the portrayal of (health) inequalities and examines each in terms of its robustness as a potential indicator or measure. It aims to provide:

- A brief definition and overview of the category.
- Brief evidence of a health-related association.
- A brief discussion of some of the problems of interpretation.
- Summary and recommendations for using the category as a guide to inequalities.
- Principal data sources associated with the category.

General problems with categories and classification

Despite a long history of defining social groups since the 1800s and the work of Karl Marx, there is little consistency and clarity in the concepts and measures used. In particular:

- The wide variety of indexes of social position are often difficult to interpret.
- Few reviews systematically examine all (or even several) social positions in connection with health; and even fewer address the potential influence of different variables (e.g. sex, marital status, ethnicity, occupation and area of residence) upon one another.

Moreover, the relationship between social disadvantage and ill health is complex, the definition of 'health' is rarely made explicit and there are competing definitions (Box 2).

Box 2

Blaxter [10], based on interview material, shows that we should distinguish between at least five different definitions of health:

1. Existence or absence of chronic *disease*.
2. *Illness* – freedom from illness not as a present state, but as a frequent occurrence.
3. *Function* or the consequence of health status, often considered in terms of disability.
4. Physical *unfitness/fitness*.
5. Psycho-social ill health or *malaise*.

Last, many forms of disadvantage related to ill health are themselves inter-correlated (for example, being non-white, working in an unskilled occupation living in the inner city, being the female head of a single parent family) and disaggregating these components may be misleading. Indeed, individuals simultaneously occupy a position on several dimensions, so that the interactions between these may have important consequences (Box 3).

Box 3

Example

A teenage Pakistani woman living in Bradford and married to a self-employed shopkeeper cannot be understood solely in terms of her age, ethnicity, gender, area of residence, occupational class, or household. The influence that all these different socio-cultural and demographic categories have upon one another crucially affect her life chances, albeit in ways that are difficult to measure.

The subtlety of these axes of social differentiation in relation to health are seldom well studied, even by sociologists; and constitute pitfalls for anyone using only one classifier. A thorough examination of the processes connecting a particular social position with health can produce useful insights about linkages between other social positions and health. The testing of resulting hypotheses can clarify and refine knowledge about the specificity or generaliseability of the processes involved.

Categorisations which may be used to define health inequalities

Three broad groups of categorisations are generally employed in the literature and in the arena of public debate upon inequalities, although differentiation between them is rarely explicit:

- Social demography (age, area of residence, sex and ethnicity/ race).
- Social and economic status (car ownership, employment, income, occupational social class, socio-economic groupings, tenure status).
- Social environment (housing conditions, social networks, social support).

We shall slightly refine the groups by distinguishing explicitly, first between:

- Demographic variables (age, sex).
- Socio-demographic categories (area of residence, ethnicity).

and second between:

- Measures of economic status.
- Measures of social position.

and finally between:

- Social environment, including housing conditions, rural versus urban.
- Social capital, including social networks and social supports.

2.2 The Proposed Categories

2.2.1 Demographic

The demographic categories of age and sex are known to be strongly associated with morbidity and mortality, although the differences between age groups, and between men and women, are not normally seen as an inequity (whilst differences between men and women in terms of employment and income are seen as inequitable and, to a certain extent, the same is true for differences between generations). In geographical terms, however, the age category may be a useful measure for highlighting where one might expect peaks and troughs in health and morbidity in a given region or area. For example, high numbers of residential care homes, or concentrations of people of retirement age, or of young children may signal potential need for access to health and social care. Where age groups are more evenly distributed in a given region or population, this would not be such a useful measure by itself. The sexes are normally quite evenly spread within communities (exceptions include sex-specific schools, care homes, monastic communities or prisons).

Age

Age is a clearly defined and easily measured category in western industrialised societies.

Examples of age-related health associations [11]

- Death rates are relatively high up to four years of age, then decrease up to later childhood.
- In men, the death rate rises abruptly in late adolescence and continues to rise thereafter, whilst in women there is a more gradual increase.
- Causes of death are different at different ages.
- Self-reported chronic illness increases steadily with age (Table 2.l).
- Height varies with age, both cross-sectionally and, for any given cohort (groups that are born during a particular year of group of years), over time.
- Blood pressure tends to rise with age in individual societies.

Table 2.1. *Proportion reporting long-term illness by sex by age*

%	*Up to 14*	*15–34*	*35–54*	*55–64*	*65–74*	*75–84*	*85+*
Men	24	25	39	54	72	79	75
Women	22	28	39	56	69	72	78

Source: Health Survey for England, 2000.

However, interpreting age gradients is more problematic because some apparent associations may be due to:

- Period effects (what happened during a particular year or decade).
- Cohort effects (the experience of that group born during a particular year or group of years).
- The process of ageing itself.
- The social as well as physiological aspects of growing older.

Moreover, there has been an upward trend in the reporting of sickness, such that twice as many 45–64 year olds are now claiming that their activity has been restricted in the last fortnight (Table 2.2).

Table 2.2. *Trends in self-reported sickness for 45–64-year-olds (1972–1998)*

%	*1972*	*1981*	*1991*	*1998*
Long-term illness	30	41	41	44
Limiting long-term illness	23	26	29	28
Restricted activity in last 14 days	9	12	13	19
Reporting general health as 'not good'	12	12	12	14

Source: General Household Survey Living in Britain, ONS, 2001.

Only well-designed prospective studies can disentangle these different effects (Section 10).

Sex

Nearly all health data are differentiated at origin by sex. The assumption that there will be distinctive profiles for each sex means that most social and health data are presented and analysed separately. Indeed, there is a relative lack of systematic comparison or attempts to account for the differences between the sexes, whether in terms of gender or anything else.

It is worth noting, routine health and social statistics data are rarely collected for different gender orientations (such as transsexual) or for sexuality (homosexual or lesbian), and, when they are, it is often difficult to believe them.

Examples of sex-related health associations

- Mortality in men is higher than in women throughout the life course so that women have a longer life expectancy.
- Causes of death differ, with men more likely to die of circulatory disease and women of cancer.
- Women are more likely to be diagnosed as suffering from psychosomatic conditions and manic depressive psychosis.
- On average, men are taller than women from the age of 15 (Table 2.3) [11].

Table 2.3. *Height (cm) by sex by age*

	Up to 14	*15–34*	*35–54*	*55–64*	*65–74*	*75–84*	*85+*
Men	130.2	176.4	175.1	172.9	170.9	168.1	165.0
Women	129.9	162.9	162.2	160.1	157.8	154.5	151.3

Source: Health Survey for England, 2000.

Summary and recommendations

The demographic categories of both age and sex may be a useful initial guide to potential health status and risk, as:

- Both age and sex are strongly related to health outcomes.
- Age and sex are relatively easy to define and measure in any given community.

But, they are rarely sufficient on their own. Whilst the over-representation, or presence of concentrations of a particular age-group in a community (high numbers of children or elderly) may be a useful guide to that community's health inequalities and needs, sex is not as useful. In general, age and sex alone are too specific to be used as inequality measures without additional categories, to indicate disadvantage.

Data sources

The Decennial Censuses are the main source of information on the age–sex composition of the U.K. population. Apart from national and regional figures, counts are available for the two main tiers of local authorities and electoral wards (postcode sectors in Scotland). The 2001 Census produced a new low-level area base, standard output areas (SOAs) (Census material is available via the ONS website – see Section 8 for more details). In the years between Censuses, estimates of the age–sex populations of local authorities and larger areas are released annually, based on projections from the last Census. A large number of sources are used in calculating these estimates, including birth and death rates, figures on immigration, emigration and mobility, and data on the numbers and location of students and armed forces. There have been concerns that such projections may be less accurate for certain population groups; for example, students and older people. The ONS Neighbourhood Statistics site holds several alternative sets of population estimates by electoral wards.

The registration lists of general practices are the main alternative source of information to the Census on population, age and sex. The Department of Health has produced counts for its administrative areas based on general practice lists and also counts for ward populations. Because of concerns of 'list inflation and deflation', both sets of counts have been reconciled to local authority level Census projections. The figures are available via the Compendium of Clinical and Health Indicators, currently only to people in the NHS, but there are plans to extend the access.

Because age and sex differentiation is so pervasive, researchers frequently standardise data for age and sex before analysing their data to explore the effects of the dimensions (e.g. ethnicity, area of residence). It is important to emphasise that this is not a foolproof procedure (see Section 3.1 for further discussion).

- Where data is standardised using age groups (the usual procedure), there may still be within-group age-related effects. This is particularly a problem among older age groups (e.g. 75+). The alternative – to adjust for age as a continuous variable – is usually impossible because of insufficient data.
- Whether standardisation is carried out in terms of age as a grouped or continuous variable, the presumption is that age and sex have additive or sometimes multiplicative effects on health. If

the joint effects of age and sex have a different functional form, then there will remain effects after standardisation.

- Several may dispute that one should always adjust for age and sex before examining other inequalities. It could be argued that ethnicity or social class are more important and therefore causally prior in the process of generating inequalities.

2.2.2 Socio-demographic Categories

In this section, we examine the socio-demographic categories of area of residence and ethnicity. Depending on the context, the categories in this section may not always be well-differentiated from those in other sections.

Area of residence

A group may be defined by the type of place of residence of its members, such as the inhabitants of a particular housing estate, or block of flats. The social value and status (including monetary value) attached to different postcodes are now well-accepted in the real estate business. For example, it is used in assessing risk of property crime in household insurance, and increasingly for other commercial or consumer purposes.

Associations between morbidity, mortality and place of residence have long been noted, with research now suggesting an independent effect of area upon the health of individuals and households within that area. The mechanism(s) through which such effects occur are, however, difficult to establish.

Moreover, present-day area boundaries more readily reflect administrative interests (electoral ward, local council, etc.) rather than 'real communities'. And these boundaries also change over time as with Census-derived areas.

<u>Examples of area-related health associations [11]</u>

- There is a gradient in mortality from low in the south and east of the country to high in the north and west. These are found for most causes of death and for all the major causes, e.g. circulatory disease, malignant neoplasms, respiratory disease, and accidents, poisonings and violence.
- People living in the south of England are taller than those living in the north.
- Blood pressure is higher in the north.

- There are variations within as well as between regions with significantly higher standardised mortality for men in inner city areas with lower quality older housing, over-spill estates, mining areas and multi-occupied and immigrant areas.

Summary and recommendations

- Associations between morbidity, mortality and place of residence have long been noted.
- Research suggests an independent effect of area upon the health of individuals and households within that area.
- The mechanisms through which such effects occur are difficult to interpret.
- Place of residence (monitored through postcode) may be a relatively sensitive measure of potential inequality and need, particularly if combined with other measures of socio-economic or demographic status.

Data sources

As for data on age and sex, the Census is the main source of the numbers of people living in a locality. In the years between Censuses, sub-local authority level population counts have been estimated (often by local authorities) from the register of electors. Though such figures are not compiled nationally, they may be available from local authorities, or agencies such as the Public Health Observatories.

GP registers provide an alternative source of population counts – see earlier section (on data sources for population age and sex) for details.

A frequently made argument is that the administrative area boundaries used in population statistics do not coincide with the boundaries of communities. In particular, there is concern that some urban electoral wards are too large and heterogeneous to provide a sensible base for analysis or social planning. For the 1991 Census, it was possible to use population counts for sub-ward areas or enumeration districts (EDs) to estimate the numbers in smaller areas. SOAs for the 2001 Census serve a similar purpose. In some, mainly inner-city, areas with high population mobility and a tendency for census under-enumeration, local authorities will make their own population estimates – often by some combination of sources, such as Council Tax returns, the Register of Electors and local surveys or censuses.

Local authorities and charities may also conduct their own censuses covering 'hard-to-reach' groups such as the homeless, who are often missed in the national Census.

Ethnicity

The recording of ethnicity has always been problematic in routine data collection, with different definitions of ethnicity in each of the 1981, 1991 and 2001 Censuses. Researchers have attempted to establish ethnicity by using names, or have carried out local or ad hoc studies, often concentrating on specific conditions affecting ethnic minority groups. The complexities are illustrated in Box 4. A more helpful approach may be to include any minority group within a nation state defined by language, nationality or origin. In any particular situation it should be possible to reach a much more precise definition. For example, in a study of the levels of drinking amongst the Irish, it was crucial to distinguish between groups defined not only on their place of birth but also on where they were currently living and on their parents' place of birth (Box 5).

Box 4

Ethnic identity

". . .ethnic identity is formed in relation to a number of dimensions: self-description, being traditional, participation in the ethnic community, and racialisation. So, rather than being something based solely on country of origin, as would be suggested by definitions of ethnicity used in earlier studies, ethnic identity can be seen to be influenced by the wider social structure. Any measure of ethnicity needs to allow for this. These analyses suggest that the relationship between ethnicity and health is also mediated by structural factors, explored here in terms of socio-economic position, and racial harassment and discrimination.

This would suggest that while traditional measures of ethnic group can allow us to recognise the existence of ethnic inequalities in health, in order to fully investigate the relationship between ethnicity and health, a more sophisticated assessment of ethnicity is required, which can both adequately account for the different forms of social disadvantage experienced by ethnic minority groups and the various ways in which racism itself can impact on physical and mental health. Racism and its accompanying social disadvantage are important aspects of the lives of people from ethnic minority groups, and this must be incorporated into strategies to address ethnic inequalities in health . . ."

Examples of ethnically related health associations

- South Asian and African born male immigrants had lower age-standardised mortality; whilst women had higher rates than the rest of the population.
- Men from Ireland have higher mortality than men in England and Wales.

Box 5

Example

Although there has been a concerted attempt to introduce ethnic monitoring in the U.K., the Irish as a group are excluded [12], despite the fact that death rates for Irish in England are high (see International Council on Migration). Ultimately this may be due to the way in which they are treated in England but the immediate cause is probably associated with their higher alcohol consumption than the English and the Irish in Ireland (Table 2.4).

Table 2.4. *Distribution between light, moderate and heavy drinking of Irish compared to British*

	Republic-Irish	*Northern-Irish*	*Republic-British*	*Northern Irish-British*	*British-British*	*Total N (100%)*	*Irish in Ireland (% distribution)*
Light	59.0	56.8	55.7	58.3	64.3	10,774	65
Moderate	28.6	31.5	33.5	25.6	27.3	4633	30
Heavy	12.3	11.7	10.9	16.1	8.4	1448	5
N	227	111	442	168	15,907	16,855	2724

Note 1: Republic-Irish: those born in the Irish Republic; Northern-Irish: those born in Northern Ireland; Republic-British: those born in Britain with one or both parents born in the Irish Republic; Northern Irish-British: those born in Britain with one or both parents born in Northern Ireland; British-British: British-born residents whose parents were also born in Britain.
Note 2: Light: up to 7 units per week for women, 10 units per week for men; Moderate: 7–25 units for women, 10–35 units for men; Heavy: over 25 units for women, over 35 units for men. Source: OPCS (1990)
Source: Harrison et al. [13].

- Early mortality in the second generation is higher.
- Low birth weight rates are higher among children born to mothers from Africa or Asia.

Table 2.5 shows the mortality rates for three different groups of causes and for suicide for different groups of immigrants. Those born in Ireland have higher rates for circulatory and respiratory diseases and for external causes, with very different rates for men and women for suicide; those born in South Asia and the African continent have higher rates only for circulatory diseases and for external causes with men having lower and women having higher rates for suicide, and men and women born in the Caribbean have different experiences for all three groups of causes, but not for suicide.

Although no one group has constantly high or low rates; the pattern defies simple description.

Table 2.5. *Standardised mortality rates for groups of diseases and suicide rates*

		Ireland	*South Asia*	*Caribbean*	*African*
All circulatory	M	117	133	77	127
	F	118	136	141	136
All respiratory	M	157	88	61	105
	F	140	104	101	106
All external causes	M	190	85	105	99
	F	59	113	100	136
Suicide	M	126	71	80	–
	F	31	149	84	–

Note: The data for the three groups of diseases, but not for suicide, are standardised by social class (on the assumption that a set of health risk factors may not apply very well to people who have spent half or two-thirds of their lives in the developing world) [11].
Source: Balarajan and Balsa [14]; Britten [15]; Raleigh and Balarajan [16].

Summary and recommendations

- Although there are some striking health and mortality associations by ethnic group, their interpretation is difficult and may be partially due to the influence of other factors.
- The recording of ethnicity has always been problematic in routine data collection, with different definitions of ethnicity in each of the 1981, 1991 and 2001 Censuses.
- Some vulnerable groups may not be recorded as an ethnic minority, and hence impossible to study through these means (e.g. the Irish).
- Ethnic association can be a useful indicator for measuring potential inequalities, however, it should be carefully applied to specific situations where it is relevant and, when possible, combined with other socio-economic and demographic measures.

Data sources

Again, the Decennial Census is the main national data source. Local surveys are quite common, and ethnic monitoring in support of equal opportunities legislation may be a further source of local information. Most of the main national surveys include questions on ethnicity, but sample sizes are too small to provide local area estimates.

Other routes that have been used to estimate the numbers in ethnic minorities in specific areas include the application of name recognition software to databases such as the electoral register and GP registration lists (the use of the latter will be restricted to GPs and health authorities with access to the lists).

Family structure and marital status

There is substantial evidence that adult health status is strongly influenced by childhood experience. Longitudinal studies of birth cohorts such as the 1946, 1958 and 1970 British Birth Cohort Studies show how a wide range of childhood factors are associated with adult health. It is assumed that most of these effects can best be captured by the socio-economic status of the household or parents, but the family or house-hold structure is also important. There are at least three possible structural dimensions:

- Household size.
- Number of adults and their age–sex breakdown, number of children and their age–sex breakdown.
- Relationship between different household members.

These can be problematic because individuals may be more or less permanent members of the household and relationships are often difficult to capture in a categorical measure. In particular, the increasing trend towards cohabitation makes "marital status" a more complicated variable to collect than previously. In Sweden, official data have not attempted to distinguish between cohabitation and marriage to the opposite sex partner, for some time. Marital status is therefore seldom used as such in analyses, although 'living alone' versus cohabitation is used.

Examples of health-associations related to marital status [11]

- Married people generally have lower death rates than single or formerly married persons.
- Births outside marriage have higher stillbirth, post-neonatal mortality and low birth weight rates.
- Married people are less likely to report long-standing chronic illness than single or formerly married persons.
- Rates of psychiatric disorder as detected by community surveys are higher among the separated and divorced than among the married.
- Blood pressure is higher among the single.
- Average height among remarried couples is lower.

Summary and recommendations

- Whilst powerful associations have been observed between marital status and health, the increasing trend towards cohabitation means that marital status is less used, instead living alone or cohabiting may be used.

- Other relationships, such as that between a teenager and his/her parents, may be important determinants of health but difficult to capture quantitatively.
- Although the family environment is recognised as having a strong influence on current and future health status, the presumption is that those effects are best captured through socio-economic status variables.

Data sources

The Decennial Census is the national data set on household composition and marital status with the greatest population coverage, but several major national surveys, such as Health Survey for England (HSE) and The General Household Survey (GHS) have more detail on household structure than the Census. Provided one is mainly interested in comparing households of different types and is not interested in controlling for local area effects, then such surveys may be preferable to the Census, and it will certainly provide more information on topics such as use of health services and income.

2.2.3 Measures of Economic Status

There is a general consensus that economic status (measured by level of income) and health outcomes are intimately related. Hence, the distribution and level of income should be a good indicator of health inequalities in a community. However, whether it is actual level of income (e.g. a 'breadline' threshold), or the relative income level (of an individual to the community average/median income level) that influences health status is still debated [17,18] (see also Section 11). This section examines the different commonly used proxy measures for income or wealth. Income is the 'gold standard' for this section, assuming that total real income can be counted, such that the proxies are evaluated by comparing their power of discrimination against that of income. Other categories that usually reflect social position independent of income and wealth are considered in the next section.

Measures of current income

Modern definitions and measurements of income and wealth are complex, attracting a commensurate literature. For example:

- There is a wide range of possible sources of income, including actual cash.
- There are usually difficulties in accounting for the distribution of income within individual households.
- Relatively simple definitions such as take-home pay are still complex because of different benefit systems, bonus systems, etc.

- Other than taxable income declared to the Inland Revenue, there is no routine recording of income.
- The reasons and extent of under-reporting vary through the income distribution.
- It is difficult to measure either income or wealth precisely in surveys because direct questioning tends to reduce the overall response rate. The usual procedure therefore is to request for an indication of the household's average income range.

Some of these points are illustrated in Table 2.6, showing what percentage of men and women in households headed by people in different social classes report different sources of income. Just over two-thirds report income from earnings, although this varies between four-fifths of those in professional households to just over half of those in unskilled manual households. It is also striking how there are diametrically opposed gradients for those reporting state benefits and investments. Similarly, there are also interesting trends/differences between men and women. Capturing income, whether through surveys or tax returns, is difficult.

Proxies for income and wealth

In addition to the measurement problems there are unpredictable fluctuations in household income over time. Economists have developed the notion of 'permanent income' to reflect the stable or long-run level of income available to a household. Given the difficulties in measurement in a survey context, a number of proxies are used instead.

Car ownership

The Census asks whether a household has one or two or more cars available. Once considered a good proxy for wealth if not for income, car ownership now has to be treated with caution as a proxy measure for the distribution of wealth, for the following reasons:

- In general, car ownership has increased greatly in recent years and across all social sectors; in particular, the decline in public transport in many areas has forced more people to use private transport, regardless of their income.
- There are difficulties of distinguishing between ownership and use of a vehicle. For example, people in employment may have the use of a company car, but not have their own car.
- Car availability depends on the number of other drivers in the household.
- Traffic congestion and parking difficulties in some central cities may cause otherwise wealthy people not to own a car.

Table 2.6. *Percentages reporting various sources of income by social class and sex*

Social class	*Sex*	*Number of persons*	*Earnings from employment or self-employment*	*State retirement pension*	*Pension from former employer*	*Child benefit*	*Other state benefits*	*Interest from savings and investments*	*Other kinds of regular allowance from outside your household*	*No source of income*
I	Men	229	81.2	17.0	21.8	28.7	7.0	41.9	7.0	0.0
Professional	Women	66	83.3	12.1	10.6	39.4	10.6	43.9	7.6	0.0
	Total	295	81.7	15.9	19.3	31.1	7.8	42.4	7.1	0.0
II	Men	1009	72.8	23.0	26.7	31.9	13.1	33.5	5.5	0.0
Managerial	Women	1034	76.6	21.3	22.5	33.6	14.6	32.3	7.6	0.1
technical	Total	2043	74.7	22.1	24.6	32.8	13.9	32.9	6.6	0.0
IIIN	Men	418	71.5	26.3	27.3	30.4	21.8	28.0	5.5	0.0
Skilled	Women	1441	67.5	26.4	22.6	36.3	26.7	24.0	4.4	0.0
non-manual	Total	1859	68.4	26.4	23.7	35.0	25.6	24.9	4.7	0.0
IIIM	Men	1105	65.2	27.3	21.9	30.8	35.7	15.7	3.3	0.1
Skilled	Women	318	55.3	35.8	24.2	33.6	50.3	14.8	4.7	0.0
manual	Total	1423	63.0	29.2	22.4	31.4	39.0	15.5	3.7	0.1
IV	Men	457	64.3	22.8	20.4	31.3	42.7	12.7	5.3	0.2
Semi-skilled	Women	723	57.8	28.2	17.7	45.6	58.5	11.8	5.0	0.1
manual	Total	1180	60.3	26.1	18.7	40.1	52.4	12.1	5.1	0.2
V	Men	133	58.6	26.3	14.3	36.1	63.2	15.0	5.3	0.0
Unskilled	Women	309	48.2	46.3	22.7	27.5	63.1	7.4	3.9	0.3
manual	Total	442	51.4	40.3	20.1	30.1	63.1	9.7	4.3	0.2
Total	Men	3395	69.1	24.4	23.4	31.4	27.1	24.0	4.8	0.1
	Women	3919	65.9	27.4	21.6	36.5	33.8	22.1	5.5	0.1
	Total	7314	67.4	26.0	22.5	34.1	30.7	23.0	5.2	0.1
		SD	46.9	43.9	41.7	47.4	65.2	42.1	22.1	2.6

Note: Other state benefits include job-seekers allowance, income support, family credit and housing benefit. Totals includes 12 armed forces (10 men and 2 women) and 60 not fully described (34 men and 26 women).
Source: Health Survey for England, Department of Health, 2000.

Some of these points are illustrated in Table 2.7, which shows the proportions reporting a long-standing illness by car availability in the household and income quintiles.

The proportions reporting a long-standing illness declines substantially from those with no cars to households with one or more cars, but the difference between those with one car and those with two or more cars is much less substantial. Whilst the proportion reporting a long-standing illness decreases from the second to the fifth quintile, the gradient is much sharper amongst those with no cars than those with two or more cars.

Table 2.7. *Long-standing illness by car availability in household by income quintiles*

	Income quintiles					
	First	*Second*	*Third*	*Fourth*	*Fifth*	*All*
No cars available	49	62	56	41	37	53
One car in household	45	50	39	33	34	39
Two cars + available	46	38	36	33	30	33
Total	47	54	40	34	32	40

Notes: Income quintile (these are adjusted for household composition): first or bottom quintile (≤£7186); second quintile (>£7186 ≤£10,834); third quintile (>£10,834 ≤£17,890); fourth quintile (>£17,890 ≤£27,705); top quintile (>£27,705).
Source: Health Survey for England, Department of Health (2000).

Council tax band

Before the community charge or 'poll tax', the rateable value of a house was a very good indication of its actual value, without requiring individual property valuations. The change to council tax has gone some way to restore the *status quo ante*. It can be used as a general proxy for relative income status, although there are several important caveats to consider:

- Every house is 'banded' from A (least) to H (greatest) according to its value; but the ranges of each band depend on the overall level of rates in the Council.
- Although in many cases the category or 'band' may afford an approximate guide of household income, people of lower income do not always occupy houses of least value, nor people with higher income occupy more affluent homes.
- Professional or other employed single people or couples without children may occupy smaller houses, particularly if 'first-time buyers'.

- Older, retired people may find it difficult or be reluctant to leave larger one-time family homes that, through size, location or both have come to be valued in the more affluent council tax bands.

Tenure status

Tenure has been another proxy measure of economic status and the simple three-fold classification of housing tenure into owner–occupiers, private renters and council home tenants, originally demonstrated to be strongly associated with mortality in the Longitudinal Study [19], is now a less sensitive indicator for a number of reasons:

- Since the widespread implementation of the 'right-to-buy' policy, a majority of households in the U.K. now own their own home.
- Mortgage debt and insecure ownership are now accepted as a serious problem for many people.
- Much private accommodation is now as expensive or more expensive to rent than to pay for a mortgage.
- Stringent procedures used in the private rental sector may operate to discriminate against people of low income or insecure employment status.
- Housing may also be provided as part of an overall employment remuneration package resulting in confusion over status, inferred income, etc.

Nevertheless compared to car ownership, there is a more consistent relationship between tenure status and reports of illness. This is illustrated in Table 2.8, looking at the proportions reporting long-standing illness by tenure status within income quintiles. The percentage reporting long-standing illness decreases from 55% for those who own outright to 31% for those buying on mortgage, and there are similar decreases for all income quintiles. In this case, the decline from second to fifth quintile is reproduced at approximately the same rate within each group. However, interpreting these gradients is complex because the values are confounded by age (as those who own outright tend to be older, except among the top income quintile, and those who are renting tend to be younger).

Summary and recommendations

Although household or individual income may be a useful guide to economic position and potential health status, the following caveats should be considered:

- Real income is difficult to estimate accurately; 'wealth' is even more difficult to define or measure.

Table 2.8. *Long-standing illness by tenure status of household by income quintiles*

	Income quintiles					
	First	*Second*	*Third*	*Fourth*	*Fifth*	*All*
Own outright	61	68	55	47	45	55
Renting	45	54	46	36	30	36
Buying on mortgage	39	40	32	30	29	31
Total	47	54	40	34	32	40

Notes: Income quintile (these are adjusted for household composition): first or bottom quintile (≤£7186); second quintile (>£7,186 ≤£10,834); third quintile (>£10,834 ≤£17,890); fourth quintile (>£17,890 ≤£27,705); top quintile (>£27,705).
Source: Health Survey for England, Department of Health (2000).

- Categories once considered as valid 'proxies' of wealth or income, such as car ownership or housing tenure, are no longer sensitive indicators of socio-economic variation owing to changes in the last 20 years.
- Thus, although, the Health Survey for England (HSE) show that there is an impact of car ownership and tenure status upon health, these tables show that one cannot assume that that there is a simple direct effect. Thus, great care needs to be taken in its interpretation.
- Whilst council tax band is less affected by these changes, it is only useful variable to indicate relative wealth *within* a single council area.
- Because of these limitations, strategies which seek to target health inequalities based upon measures of income alone may not be adequate.
- Therefore, if measures of personal income are used, other measures are also included to form a more accurate and balanced picture.

At small area level, some of these problems are attenuated especially for council tax band, although it can still only be used as an indicator of relative wealth. However, there are a multiplicity of aggregate measures of poverty (see Section 6).

Data sources

Rather unusually, at least when compared to many of the other dimensions of socio-economic classification, routine data on some aspects of low income are more widely available than data on average income itself. Thus, there is a wide range of claimant counts available but only one measure of average income.

Income and benefits

The New Earnings Survey and Index of Average Earnings are two of the major sources of information on pay and income from work. The former is based on a 1% national sample of employees whose tax is handled via Pay As You Earn (PAYE). Area analyses are available from NOMIS. The Index of Average Earnings results are available from the ONS.

Electoral ward level data on various means-tested and disability-related benefits is available from the ONS Neighbourhood Statistics website.

To be useful, these numbers should be related to ward populations. Unfortunately, the Census-based estimates are not released at sub-local authority level, so other sources must be used. Section 2.2.2 describes several possibilities, including the Index of Multiple Deprivation-2004 related ward level counts and ward level population counts computed by the Department of Health.

Data sources for proxies for income and wealth

Data on car ownership and tenure status are available from the Census at small area level. Other sources worth considering are the market research-driven classifications of areas, such as the ACORN or SuperProfile classifications. With suitable permission, or funding to purchase data, further sources include data on council tax banding (from local councils), and insurance company property valuation databases. Land registry details of average house prices, for different types of properties, are now held by local area on the ONS Neighbourhood Statistics website.

2.2.4 Measures of Social Position

Education

Educational achievement is usually considered a good guide to social position and a robust indicator of inequalities [8,20]. Education has several advantages, including:

- Level of education can be defined on the same basis regardless of level of economic activity (e.g. whether a person is 'gainfully employed' or not).
- Level of education does not generally change after youth and is not normally influenced by illness (excepting in the case of a few rare illnesses), whereas a person's occupation and income level can change as a result of health problems.
- Information on education is more comparable than information on occupational class, both internationally and over time.

Levels and distribution of education

Until recently, most of the population in Europe has received the same general level of education prescribed by compulsory schooling. Indeed, it used to be difficult to find meaningful differences in, for example, mortality, because level of education does not vary sufficiently in a given population.

In order to develop an up-to-date and useful measure of education, adaptations of earlier systems for classifying and measuring education (e.g. the three-fold classification in Valkonen et al. [8]) take account of the recent lengthening of compulsory education and the distinction between two basic educational levels:

- Compulsory schooling, including primary through secondary school up to the age of 16 years.
- Higher educational experiences, including everything beyond age 16, including vocational qualifications.

Further refinements may distinguish vocational and academic qualifications gained between the ages of 16 and 18, from higher university level qualifications. However, it becomes increasingly difficult to code all the possible educational qualifications consistently over different time periods.

The percentage reporting long-standing illness decreases from 52% for those whose head of household left school at 15 to 36% for those whose head of household left full-time education at 17 or older, but this decline is not reproduced within either the second or the top income quintile (Table 2.9). Further, there are complex interactions with age and sex, because the age of leaving compulsory schooling has been gradually increasing and recently there has been more sex equality in level of education obtained.

Table 2.9. *Long-standing illness by year of leaving full-time education of head of household by income quintiles*

	Income quintiles					
	First	*Second*	*Third*	*Fourth*	*Fifth*	*All*
Not yet finished	40	40	32	34	28	34
Left at 14 or under	70	74	73	56	53	71
15	59	66	53	45	37	52
16	47	46	38	37	32	39
17,18,19+	36	57	36	32	35	36
Total	53	61	45	37	34	44

Notes: Income quintile (these are adjusted for household composition): first or bottom quintile (≤£7186); second quintile (>£7186 ≤£10,834); third quintile (>£10,834 ≤£17,890); fourth quintile (>£17,890 ≤£27,705); top quintile (>£27,705).
Source: Health survey for England, 2000.

Summary and recommendations

Education is widely seen as a good indicator of social position and a robust indicator of inequalities. However:

- In developed industrialised nations, schooling up to a certain age has been compulsory for several decades,[2] making length of education a poor indicator for some age groups (Section 7.4).
- Level of education may be measured by qualification, which also better reflects a person's life chances (though more difficult to categorise).
- The relationship of educational attainment to geographical area may be difficult to map.

It is, therefore, probably not advisable to use education as the only classifier. When it is used, one should always control at least for age, reflecting the period during which the individual was in the school system.

Data sources

The Decennial Census provides a limited amount of data on education. It asks people aged 16 and over to list their educational attainments and records whether or not a person is a student of full-time student(s) in each household. The Census additionally includes a question on professional and vocational qualifications.

Child benefit data (from NOMIS), broken down by the age of child for those aged 16 and over, provides an indirect estimate of those staying in full-time education after the compulsory education.

The *Labour Force Survey* (from the Data Archive) collects data on adult qualifications.

Non-census sources on educational attainment (e.g. Index of Multiple Deprivation and Office of the Deputy Prime Minister (ODPM)) include data on absenteeism, mainly derived from local educational authorities, or from educational institutions. In the latter case, the catchment area has to be inferred as there are no published details of the distribution of pupil postcodes.

The compilers of the Index of Multiple Deprivation use computerised mapping and spatial data analytical systems (Geographical Information Systems – GIS) to approximate ward maps of primary school catchment areas. This method is unlikely to be valid for the much larger and complicated secondary school areas. There may also be difficulties accurately inferring primary school catchment areas in parts of large towns and cities using GIS. Nevertheless, this is a unique source and the Index of Multiple Deprivation 2004 ward level estimates of *primary school pupils at*

---

[2] For example, although it is now age 16 in the U.K., it was 14 immediately after the second World War, and successively raised to 15, then 16.

Key stage 2 (for summer, 2002) are available on the ONS Neighbourhood Statistics site.

Local school-based data together with additional 'local knowledge' may afford a more accurate inference of catchment areas than by using GIS-generated information. However, in areas where schools have very wide or socially diverse catchment areas, problems may be experienced with any method.

Postcode data may provide a simple measure of access to schools, computed from both school and pupil postcodes. Both child benefit data and GP registrations are sources for such data, but may be difficult to obtain.

The Universities and Colleges Admissions service keeps postcoded records of university applicants with details of the outcome of the application. For the Index of Multiple Deprivation 2004, they were prepared to release data on the numbers per ward whose applications were successful. Ward level university admissions data can be found on the ONS Neighbourhood Statistics site.

Employment status

An important measure of social position (as well as a guide to income) may be a person's employment status, that is whether or not they are 'gainfully employed'. The link between unemployment and social disadvantage, is generally accepted with the current socio-economic configuration [21]. Whether or not a person is employed may influence their well being and ability to stay healthy, but the way these categories have been defined, and therefore how sensitive they are as potential measures, in most publicly available datasets is problematic.

Definition of employment and unemployment

The International Labour Organisation's (ILO) 1982 definition of employment, agreed upon at the Thirteenth International Conference of Labour Statisticians (ICLS [22]), states that the 'employed' comprise all persons above the age specified for measuring the economically active population who, during a specified (brief) period (usually one week or one day), were in one of the following categories:

- Paid employment: 'at work' or 'with a job but not at work'.
- Self-employment: 'at work': persons who performed some work for profit or family gain, in cash or in kind.
- 'With an enterprise but not at work'.

The notion of 'some work' in self-employment only needs to be work for at least *one hour*.

The conventional and most widely used definition for unemployment was originally agreed upon at the same 1982 ILO conference, and sets three criteria for clarifying people as unemployed. They should be above the age specified for measuring the economically active population and, during a specified (brief) period, should be:

- Without work.
- Available for work during the reference period.
- Actively seeking work, that is, they must have taken specific steps in quest of a job during a specified recent period.

Employment and unemployment are considered to be mutually exclusive, therefore persons engaged in any casual work at all, however small, while seeking employment are still classified as employed. The other two criteria of the definition of unemployment, 'current availability for work' and 'seeking work' aim to distinguish people who would be gainfully employed if they could find employment from people who are not actually seeking paid work (e.g. carers of young children based at home).

Rates of unemployment will clearly vary depending upon which definition is used. For example, the U.S. Bureau of Labor Statistics (BLS) has published seven alternative measures for unemployment since 1976. In 1989, the unemployment rate in the U.S. therefore varied between 1.2% and 7.9% depending upon which measure was used [23].

Under-employment

Unemployment, therefore, is a *relatively* straightforward concept, employment is more complex, as it represents a broad spectrum of working circumstances. It includes people who, though classified as 'with work', may also be looking for further gainful employment for various reasons. This group may be regarded as under-employed.

The 1966 International Congress of Labour Statistics resolution defines under-employment as "when a person's employment is inadequate, in relation to specified norms of alternative employment, account being taken of his occupational skill (training and work experience)" (ICLS, 1966). Two principal forms of under-employment are distinguished:

- 'Visible' under-employment, reflecting an insufficiency in the volume of employment.
- 'Invisible' under-employment, characterised by low income, under-utilisation of skill, low productivity and other factors.

'Visible' under-employment is defined as a sub-category of employment. There are three criteria for identifying those who are visibly under-employed:

- Working less than normal duration.
- Doing so on an involuntary basis.
- Seeking or being available for additional work during the reference period.

To measure 'invisible' under-employment, whether in respect of income, levels of skill or productivity, thresholds have to be established below which:

- The income is considered abnormally low.
- The skill is under-utilised.
- The productivity is insufficient.

Informal sector employment

The informal sector has played a growing role over the past three decades, in particular in developing countries for its role in absorbing large numbers of unskilled labour in a dualistic economy. In developed countries, however, the labour surplus is smaller and social protection systems exist, therefore the informal sector that does exist (e.g. small-scale units outside the formal economy or services rendered by one household to another) is relatively small. For practical reasons, mainly the difficulties in quantification, it is not considered further here.

Employment status is strongly associated with income (Table 2.10). However, apart from those 'in employment', the association is not straightforward.

Table 2.10. *Percentage in each income quintile by economic status*

	Income quintiles				
	First	*Second*	*Third*	*Fourth*	*Fifth*
In employment	4.5	7.3	22.0	28.6	37.6
ILO unemployed	32.8	14.2	20.7	11.1	21.1
Retired	17.2	33.6	25.4	14.0	9.8
Other economically inactive	31.1	25.7	19.8	11.7	11.7
	898	1104	1499	1464	1781
	13.3	16.4	22.2	21.7	26.4

Note: Income quintile (these are adjusted for household composition): Bottom quintile (≤£7186); second quintile (>£7186 ≤£10,834); third quintile (>£10,834 ≤£17,890); fourth quintile (>£17,890 ≤£27,705); top quintile (>£27,705).
Source: Health survey for England, 2000.

The percentage reporting long-standing illness increases from 31% for those whose head of household is in employment to 68% for those whose head of household is retired; but this is not true for all of the income quintiles. (Table 2.11). There is no consistent decline from second to fifth quintile for those in employment or unemployed by the ILO definition.

Table 2.11. *Long-standing illness by economic status of head of household by income quintiles*

	Income quintiles					
	First	*Second*	*Third*	*Fourth*	*Fifth*	*All*
In employment	32	33	32	32	32	31
ILO unemployed	31	33	39	33	22	31
Other economically inactive	61	69	58	48	46	59
Retired	68	75	66	61	57	68
Total	54	61	45	37	34	44

Notes: Income quintile (these are adjusted for household composition): first or bottom quintile (≤£7186); second quintile (>£7186 ≤£10,834); third quintile (>£10,834 ≤£17,890); fourth quintile (>£17,890 ≤£27,705); top quintile (>£27,705).
Source: Health survey for England, 2000.

Summary and recommendations

Although employment status can be a useful guide to social position, the following caveats should be considered:

- Employment is a very broad term and may include many categories of semi-employed, under-employed or otherwise low-waged earners.
- Unemployment is more explicitly defined and measured, but excludes many people who are in receipt of a low income or otherwise actively seeking more or better-paid employment.
- Strategies which seek to target health inequalities based upon measures of employment status alone may not be adequate.
- It is therefore recommended that if measures of employment status are used, additional measures are also included to form a more accurate and balanced picture.

Whilst many of these problems are attenuated at a small area level, the nature of the employment market and thus employment also varies substantially.

Data sources

Unemployment benefit claimant counts presented in various forms are available down to ward level on the ONS NOMIS website. The main options are counts (age and duration of unemployment), seasonally adjusted counts, unadjusted counts – with corresponding rates for each. The same set of options are available for claimant flows and there is an additional data set of claimant 'off-flows' showing the reason for ceasing being a claimant, the claimant's age, and duration of the most recent claim.

The Labour Force Survey provides an alternative estimate of unemployment independent of the frequent changes in the criteria for claiming unemployment benefit. It is a quarterly sample survey which collects information on personal circumstances and employment status. The full data sets are lodged with the Data Archive; a subset of recent data is available on-line from NOMIS.

The *Annual Employment Survey* replaced the annual *Census of Employment* in late 1995. This survey of approximately 130,000 businesses collects information on the nature of the business, the gender of employees, the types of jobs and whether they are full or part-time. Data are produced by ward with considerable detail on the type of business activity. It is available on-line from NOMIS, but there is a special registration procedure for this data set which requires a statement of intended use.

Other relevant data sets held by NOMIS include details of job centre vacancies, by occupation and industry, but most of these are only available at unitary authority level or higher.

Social class

Occupational social class was first introduced in 1911 by the then Registrar General as a systematic approach to classifying individuals according to their wealth (Box 6). This classification, though modified at nearly every Census since then (and thus losing its original theoretical basis), is still used as a generic measure for discriminating life chances, particularly in terms of death rates, more generally known as 'standardised mortality ratios' (SMRs). Given the origin and the ad hoc nature of the modifications, the extent to which changes in the occupational social class classification reflect the considerable changes in the occupational class structure since 1911 is unknown. Therefore, whether or not individual social class actually reflects real differences in individuals' lives and relative prosperity now is an open question. Without a detailed interview survey over several time periods including both cohort and cross-sectional components, it is impossible to document such changes. The comparison of SMRs between occupational social classes can often mask the nature of the discrimination between groups that are relevant in public health terms.

Box 6

Occupational social class and the 1911 Census

Stevenson [24] introduced the classification primarily for the analysis of fertility and infant mortality. He said, "the ideal method would classify individuals, not whole populations, by their degree of prosperity", but "doubts the value of income data even if it were routinely collected in Britain as it may fail altogether as an indicator of culture, probably the more important influence".

A number of other classifications have been introduced since the 1960s. The most well known is SEGs. This is described in the 1991 Census User's Guide as "a non-hierarchical classification which uses both occupation and employment status and aims to bring together people with jobs of similar social and economic status" [25]. It has 17 main divisions, including 'personal service workers', 'junior non-manual workers' and 'professional workers: self-employed'.

Nevertheless, despite radical modifications to the social class classification in 1991 making it almost impossible to understand what dimensions of social or economic differentiation were actually being captured, it continued to dominate. A review commissioned for the 2001 Census, kept the social class classification, but with a new set of groupings.

This new formulation for the 2001 Census is the National Statistics Socio-Economic Classification (NS-SeC). It is occupation-based and intended to give an indication of socio-economic position. It is quasi-hierarchical and replaces both the previous classifications into class and SEG (Box 7).

Box 7

NS-SeC

- Class 1 higher managerial and professional occupations (six sub-groups).
- Class 2 lower managerial and professional (six sub-groups).
- Class 3 intermediate occupations (four sub-groups, includes intermediate clerical and administrative, intermediate engineering and several other sub-groups).
- Class 4 small employers and own account workers (four sub-groups, includes some non-professional groups and some agricultural workers).
- Class 5 lower supervisory and technical occupations (three sub-groups).
- Class 6 semi-routine occupations (seven sub-groups).
- Class 7 routine occupations (five sub-groups).
- Class 8 never-worked and long-term unemployed.

Full-time students are excluded from the classification.

More details of this classification can be found in the Manual of Output Classifications for the 2001 Census, which is available on the National Statistics website.

The 2001 Census also presents its results by 'social grade', using an algorithm developed by the market research society for re-classifying the Census material. This scheme is widely used in market research, but rarely in academic work. There are six main categories:

A. Professional.
B. Middle managers.
C1. All other non-manual workers.
C2. All skilled manual workers.
D. All semi-skilled and unskilled manual workers.
E. On benefit/unemployed.

Examples of occupational social class-related health associations [11]

Despite these many caveats, the associations documented below, years ago, are still largely correct.

- There are consistent gradients by occupational class with death ratios increasing from managerial and professional occupations to unskilled labourers for both men and women.
- Occupational class of father is associated with chances of survival in the perinatal period.
- There are gradients for both chronic and acute illness by occupational class.
- Heights of children and of adults vary systematically by class.

The extent to which the current social class classification has departed from income in its capacity to discriminate health outcomes is illustrated in Table 2.12. There is a steady, although small, increase in the percentage reporting long-standing illness from 35% for those whose head of household is in Social Classes I or II to 45% for those whose head of household is in Social Classes IV or V. But this is not reflected within any of the income quintiles; and the decline from second to fifth quintile in the whole sample is not reproduced for the top two

Table 2.12. *Long-standing illness by Registrar General's occupation social class by income quintile*

	Income quintiles					
	First	*Second*	*Third*	*Fourth*	*Fifth*	*All*
I and II	44	52	37	32	32	35
III NM	42	54	52	34	35	43
III M	54	56	37	36	32	43
IV and V	46	54	43	39	22	45
Total	48	54	41	34	32	40

Notes: Income quintile (these are adjusted for household composition): bottom quintile (≤£7186); second quintile (>£7186 ≤£10,834); third quintile (>£10,834 ≤£17,890); fourth quintile (>£17,890 ≤£27,705); top quintile (>£27,705).
Source: Health survey for England, 2000.

social class groups. Whatever social class reflects, it is something very different from income.

Summary and recommendations

Occupational social class is widely seen as a good indicator of social position. However:

- The use of SMRs as a measure with social class categorisations have been demonstrated to be problematic for a number of reasons.
- Society has changed greatly since the introduction of the classification in 1911, so that it may no longer be a sensitive indicator in its present form.

Data sources

In theory, individual level data from the 2001 Census could be used to generate a suite of other measures of social position that are more relevant to current socio-economic structures, however, the main measures that are being provided are the reformulated version of social class and the market research classification: social grade.

2.2.5 Overview of Measures

A large number of different possible socio-economic characteristics of individuals have been discussed in addition to age and sex. Table 2.13 provides a brief summary and references.

Table 2.13. *Measures used to define social position*

Measure	*References*
Occupation	[26–33]
Education level	[34–37]
Income	[38,39]
Measures of material assets/wealth	[40–42]
Composite indexes: e.g. occupation, education and income	[43,44]
Economic status during childhood/father's occupation	[45–49]
Relative economic position within society	[50,51]
Community characteristics/census block or small area data	[52–61]
Measures of social structure (family structure, marital status)	[62–64]
Measures of control at work/psycho-social factors on the job	[65–67]
Deprivation	[68–74]
Position in relations of production (class position)	[75,76]
Descriptions of actors in a social movement	[77,78]

2.3 Features of the Social Environment that Might Lead to Inequalities

The classifications considered in the previous section are all characteristics of the individual or the household that are portable in the sense that they are independent of the physical and socio-economic environment (even though the salience or interpretation of, for example, car ownership, may not be). But several aspects of the physical and social environment, such as housing conditions, rural or urban residence, or social capital, can influence health differentially. These are considered together in this section.

2.3.1 Measurement of Housing Conditions

Following the Florence Nightingale proposal that "the connection between health and the dwellings of the population is one of the most important that exists" and in accordance with recent WHO definitions of acceptable housing standards in relation to health and well being (WHO 1993), housing conditions may be used as a measure for highlighting potential health inequalities.

'Poor housing'

Poor housing is usually defined in terms of overcrowding, damp and mould, indoor pollutants and infestation, cold and homelessness, including the occupation of temporary accommodation.

Whilst it is certainly the case that the impact of several of these dimensions are contingent on climate (e.g. prevalence of cold, damp and mould) or culture (e.g. what constitutes over crowding), there is a substantial corpus of research from developed western countries linking these to poor health outcomes (Table 2.14). A key issue here is *relative inequality* – subjective experiences of poor housing, overcrowding and lack of privacy compared with accepted national average standards and which may therefore be demonstrated to have detrimental effects on health indicators.

Apart from poor housing, type of housing may also be associated with adverse health consequences. High-rise accommodation and its association with health problems, in particular, has attracted criticism in the U.K. This may, in part, be a cultural artefact in that Britain has developed a housing tradition of 'horizontal urban villages' rather than high-rise apartment blocks [79]. In 1964, only 7% of households in England were living in purpose-built flats (compared with over 50% in some other European countries including Sweden and France). The U.K. changed rapidly between 1969 and 1973, when more than one million people were housed in high-rise blocks following a sudden increase in demand [80]. Almost immediately following this development, research began to link high-rise buildings with stress and mental ill health in adults, as well as slow development and respiratory disease in children [81,82]. It is unclear whether it is the *form* of housing itself or the contrast with another form seen as more appropriate; or indeed its *condition* (in terms of the quality of construction) which is associated with the development of health problems.

Box 8

The WHO definition of healthy housing (WHO, 1993)

"A human habitation that is structurally sound and relatively free from accidental injury hazards, provides sufficient space for all normal household activities for all members of the family, has readily and easily available an adequate supply of potable and palatable water, has a sanitary means of collection, storage and disposal of all liquid and solid wastes, is provided with appropriate installed facilities for personal and household hygiene, is sufficiently weatherproof and watertight, provides proper protection from the elements, especially for those persons who may be particularly susceptible, for physical and/or physiological reasons to these potentially adverse environmental conditions, provides a hypothermal indoor environment which is healthful and comfortable, is free from excessive noise from both interior and exterior sources of the structure, has natural and artificial means of illumination that are safe and adequate in quality and quantity for the fulfilment of all normal household activities and functions, is free from toxic and/or noxious odours, chemicals and other air contaminants or pollutants, has adequate but not excessive solar radiation, provides adequate protection from insects and rodents which may be reservoirs and/or vectors of disease agents, and is served by the necessary and or desirable health, welfare, social, educational, cultural and protective community services and facilities".

<u>The link between poor housing and ill health</u>

What actual mechanisms influence the housing and health relationship and how does residential area play a part in this?

To derive a widely applicable 'outcome measure' to use in quantifying the impact of *poor housing* (and/or residential area) upon the health of the resident is not as straight forward as it seems. This assumes that 'the whole package of poverty, illness and social problems could be unravelled into a single long causal chain with housing as one of the early links', whereas in reality, 'residential variables (are) richly embedded in a large matrix of individual and social variables that condition and attenuate the impact of the residential environment' [83]. We are not dealing, with a simple cause and effect, but a relatively complex scenario of interactive social and psycho-social factors for which an appropriately complex data set and analytic strategy is required [84]. Currently, the data sets in the U.K. are insufficient to meet the challenge fully.

Apart from any causal pathway linking poor housing conditions to subsequent ill health, two processes tend to select for people already suffering from ill health to live in poorer quality housing:

- When there is a shrinking social housing sector and a medical priority system operates in the allocation of such housing, people with medical needs will not only be disproportionately represented, as higher quality housing stock tended to be sold under the right to buy legislation, the social housing available may also be of a poorer standard.
- Those with medical needs unable to access social housing may not be able to afford better quality housing because their ill health may compromise their earning power; and thus they will be disproportionately represented in poorer quality accommodations [85].

Table 2.14 summarises key findings associating health problems with poor housing conditions.

Table 2.14. *The consequences of 'poor' housing circumstances for physical health*

Housing circumstance	*Consequence*	*Relevant studies*
Overcrowding	Increased risk of infectious or respiratory disease	[86]
	Reduced stature	
Damp and mould	Respiratory problems, e.g. wheezing	[87]
	Asthma, rhintis and alveolitis	[88]
	Eczema	[89–98]
Indoor pollutants and infestation	Asthma	[99–102]
Cold	Diminished resistance to respiratory infection	[103,104]
	Hypothermia	[105]
	Broncohspasm	
	Ischaemic heart disease, myocardial infarction and strokes	[106]
Homelessness-rooflessness	Problems resulting from facing the elements without protection	[107,108]
Homelessness-temporary accommodation	Problems resulting from overcrowding, noise, inadequate cooking and washing facilities	[109]

Source: OPCS (1990) and Harrison et al. [13].

Summary and recommendations

- The relationship between housing and health has long been held important.
- The mechanisms that link poor housing with ill health are not as clear or straightforward as they seem and a direct causal pathway is hard to demonstrate.
- Strategies that seek to target health inequalities based upon housing measures alone may not be adequate.
- It is recommended that additional measures be included to form a more accurate and balanced picture.

Data sources

Apart from the Census, very little information on housing is available at sub-local authority level. There are several national surveys, but samples are too small for sub-LA breakdowns. It is possible to *model* down the survey results, for example in the Index of Multiple Deprivation 2004 and Welsh Deprivation Indexes.

Level of occupancy

- The Census questions on numbers of people in the household and the number of rooms occupied are used to compute a measure of overcrowding, e.g. the numbers of households (and persons in households) living at more than 1 and more than 1.5 persons per room. This calculation periodically changes, as different types of rooms (for example, bathrooms and kitchen) are included in the denominator.

Housing amenities

- Both the 1991 and 2001 Censuses asked whether households have exclusive use of a bath or shower and of a toilet and whether there is central heating. The level of detail has been reduced for 2001, so there may be circumstances in which indicators based on the 1991 classification cannot be computed for 2001.

Physical condition of housing

The main sources on the structural condition of housing are two surveys and local authority returns.

- The English House Condition Survey (there are parallels for Wales and Scotland) includes a professional assessment of physical condition and a valuation, as well as an interview with the residents. It is based on a sample of 25,000 dwellings and is repeated every five years. Half of the properties in the 1991 survey were reassessed in 1995 in order to record any changes. The data sets are available from the ODPM.

- The ODPM conducts a second national survey, the Survey of English Housing. This survey emphasizes the type of accommodation, tenure, the experiences of the household in finding accommodation and moving, and their views of the accommodation and residential area. The survey is repeated annually and is based on a sample of 20,000 households.
- Local authority returns for the Housing Investment Programme (HIP) gives some data on housing stock, vacancies, lettings and homelessness. More specific information is provided by local authority returns on the numbers of unfit dwellings and the reason for their being 'unfit'.
- The Housing Needs Index is another LA level data source. It is based on data from the Survey of English Housing, the General Households Survey and the English House Condition Survey.

Housing tenure

The four basic categories are own outright, own on mortgage, social renting (from either the council or a housing association), and private renting. However, there are several other smaller categories that can be important in specific situations such as tied cottages in farming areas.

There are several sources relating to particular types of tenure:

- Although the Survey of English Housing collects information on tenure, the Census is the main source. The 1991 Census asked if rented accommodation was furnished or unfurnished. In 2001, this question was only asked in Scotland.
- Housing association statistics (collated by the ODPM by LA) give details of the numbers of lettings and new lettings, and a considerable range of information on the tenants.
- Local authority housing performance indicators, from OPDM, will also have some information on tenure.

2.3.2 The Urban–Rural Split and Health

Rural living in the U.K., often pictured as idyllic and second country homes for the urban elite, has been associated with higher levels of poverty and ill health in many regions [110,111]. As sparsely populated regions where the population is less nucleated than in urban contexts, they have a higher cost of access to services than urban regions [112]. Adequate provision of healthcare and other services in rural areas, therefore, usually requires deliberate policies of care or service providers.

The Lifestyles in Rural England study also investigated the composition of those households in or on the margins of poverty using the Townsend

Index. Households with just one or two elderly people were groups experiencing poverty in many of the areas surveyed, with many still having to rely on state pensions for their lifestyle needs.

> **Box 9**
>
> **Lifestyles in Rural England**
>
> The Lifestyles in Rural England study has done much to refocus attention on the nature and extent of rural poverty. Cloke et al. conclude that, "Our study shows that there is, at an aggregate level, a very important problem of low incomes and poverty in many, if not most, rural areas in England." [110]

What is meant by rural?

A definition of rural would seem useful for the purposes of research and policy making. However, the concept of 'rural' is influenced by various dimensions, such as cultural differences, employment patterns, geographical isolation and so on. Some rural communities may actually have more in common with urban communities with similar employment patterns, than with other rural areas. Population density, land use and remoteness are also important factors [113,79].

> **Box 10**
>
> **Definitions of 'rural'**
>
> A common definition is areas with low population density [112]. The OPCS definition, is simply the residual of the definition of urban areas and in effect, covers settlements of up to 1000 persons [114]. On this basis, the population of rural England is just over 4.3 million; if settlements up to 5000 persons are included then it increases to nearly 7.5 million (Rural Development Commission, 1989). The U.S. Census Bureau defines as rural those persons living in open country, on farms or in towns of fewer than 2500 people [115]. Using population size has the advantage of simplicity, but its specificity may be open to criticism; for example, some inner city areas have low resident populations.
>
> Accessibility to services is another approach to defining rurality or remoteness. The Trent Regional Helath Authority (RHA) defined as rural those communities which could not reach out-patient clinics and back in half-a-day (Trent Regional Health Authority, 1991).

Box 11

An example

One extreme example of accessibility is in Orkney, the Shetland Islands and the Western Islands off the coast of Scotland. In order to provide healthcare services, they receive the Special Islands Needs Allowance (SINA) to reflect the increased cost of (or arising from):

- Delivery of services.
- Travel costs (including lost staff time).
- Staff and goods and services.
- Lack of competition.
- Democratic and fixed management structures.
- Extreme weather conditions.

It is important to distinguish between the various ways in which population distribution might affect accessibility. SINA calibrated the difficulty of movement within and between islands in any one group using a ratio of the land area and coastline length compared with an efficient area (i.e. a circle of the same area). Clearly, this approach is only feasible for wholly island administrations; it is unlikely to be appropriate for land areas where the variation according to the shape of the boundary are unlikely to be large.

Example of rural related health associations [116]

- A study of regional differences in mental health found that north–south differences in psychiatric morbidity were less marked within urban areas than in rural areas.

Summary and recommendations

- Different studies have demonstrated relatively high rates of poverty for many rural areas.
- Careful consideration should be given to the definition of rural when undertaking research or interpreting research results.
- The main approaches used in defining rurality are:
  - population density
  - patterns of settlement
  - perceptions of population groups
  - access

- Rural areas may be more diverse than urban areas and there is a distinction between different types of rural settings. An affluent village in the south east commuter belt is quite different from an isolated Cumbrian village.
- The scale at which a definition is applied will have implications for the interpretation of data on rural areas.
- Some wards may include both rural and urban areas; and significant population heterogeneity may be present at a district or even ward level.

Data sources

There has been much effort to derive a measure of rurality driven largely by the need for a variable that can be used to divert resources to cover additional costs of public service delivery in rural areas.

These are three of the major approaches:

- Population density.
- Patterns of settlement.
- Rural occupations.

Population density can be calculated at a ward level from Census population counts and ward areas available from ONS. However, it does not reflect actual patterns of settlement and hence has a similar value for an area in which the entire population was based in a small town, and one in which the population was more evenly, but sparsely, distributed. A number of measures to address access to and ease of provision of services have either been developed, or are in the process of development. In the older and simpler versions, derived from the Census, the measure was a version of "what proportion of an area's population lived in wards above a certain density". More recent versions take account of distance from centres of population or 'settlements'. The Welsh Assembly has commissioned a major programme to produce such measures, but as yet there is not a publicly available ward level settlement measure for either England or Wales. It may be worth trying the Public Health Observatories to see if anything has been developed locally.

With the 2001 Census results, it is possible to use the data on occupational and industrial classifications to measure rurality by the proportion of people employed in agriculture, or in specific types of agricultural occupations. Opinions differ on the utility of such measures. On the one hand, they may be useful in comparing the health and conditions of those in predominately agricultural areas with those in other areas, but may be less successful in capturing those aspects of sparsity and settlement that are of interest to organisations delivering services in rural areas.

2.3.3 Social Capital

There is a long tradition of relating characteristics of different types of community to the individual's health. For example, Durkheim [117] showed how rate of suicide varied between Protestant and Catholic communities and formulated the concept of anomie to account for those variations. Whilst still used (albeit with a rather different meaning) in social psychology, the concept has fallen out of favour in social analysis, replaced by socio-political and materialist explanations. Recent reincarnations of that line of argument have been termed 'social capital'. There is no widely accepted definition, but the term refers to features of social organisation that act as resources available to individuals through membership of social networks or communities [118] that facilitate individual and collective action. Trust in others, norms of reciprocity (the expectation that a favour will be returned), and the quantity and quality of social interaction are important components of social capital. Network membership tends to lead to increased access to information and to increased possibilities of informal social control [119].

For Putnam the level of social capital in society can be measured by indicators such as the level of membership in voluntary associations of all kinds, the extent of interpersonal trust between citizens, and their perceptions of the availability of mutual aid [120,121]. But there are competing definitions [122,123]. Despite the lack of agreement on definition, researchers in health have pursued the possibility that social capital is conducive to health. Most agree that:

- Social capital is a collective dimension of society external to the individual.
- Social capital is a feature of the social structure not of the individual actors within the social structure; it is an ecological characteristic.

The argument is that social capital can be distinguished from the concepts of social networks and support, which are seen to be attributes of individuals. The different ways in which the concept has been used are shown in Table 2.15.

General evidence

The first quantitative work investigating the relationship between social capital and health was in the U.S.:

- Neighbourhoods with greater social control and social cohesion were found to have lower homicide rates [124].
- Fewer behavioural and emotional problems in childhood were found in neighbourhoods with higher church attendance and neighbourhood support [125].

Table 2.15. *Concepts used in the measurement of neighbourhood cohesion*[a]

	Hunter [126]	*Riger [127]*	*Unger [128]*	*Buckner [129]*	*Perkins [130]*
Social interaction; casual interaction (e.g. number of people you can recognise on your block: number of people who live on this block that you know by name)		✔	✔		
Frequency that you chat with neighbours	✔			✔	
Frequency that you will visit informally in neighbour's home: number of people who have a neighbourly relationship with	✔		✔	✔	
Social support (e.g. socio-emotional support)			✔	✔	✔
Instrumental support	✔		✔	✔	✔
Informational support	✔		✔	✔	✔
Social networks (e.g. personal networks (both within and outside neighbourhood))			✔	✔	
Neighbourhood social networks (e.g. neighbourhood groups)			✔		
Affective bonds sense of mutual aid (e.g. feeling that you can rely on your neighbours; believing that potential help is available)			✔		
Sense of community (e.g. membership, influence, sharing of values and emotional connection)	✔	✔		✔	
Attachment to place (e.g. plan to remain a resident of this neighbourhood for a number of years; would be sad if one had to move from this neighbourhood)		✔		✔	
Number of items	13	6	10	18	10
Reliability	NR	$\alpha = 0.56–0.59$	$\alpha = 0.88$	$\alpha = 0.95$	$\alpha = 0.76$
Validity	NR	2 Factor analysis	NR	Criterion $p < 0.001$	NR

[a] The dimensions of neighbouring are based on Unger and Wundersmann [131]. The cognitive component of neighbouring described in Unger and Wundersmann [131] is not shown because no studies measured this component.

Source: Table 3 in Lochner et al. [132].

NR, not reported.

Some work in the U.K. points to a role for social capital:

- Suicide rates are greater in areas with higher proportions of single person households, unmarried persons, private renters and movers in the last year [133].
- Enjoying living in the neighbourhood, high reciprocity, and higher levels of community activity are associated with better self-rated health for women, although not for men.

Some studies have produced contrasting findings:

- Neighbourhood social cohesion (covering attraction to the neighbourhood, whether neighbours help each other out, and sense of community) in four areas in Glasgow was not related to self-rated health, but it was associated with psychiatric morbidity (measured on the GHQ12) and with the presence of symptoms (including malaise and physical symptoms);
- Work in Luton found that some measures of social capital, such as a high level of local identity, were actually associated with poorer health [134].

HSE 2000 tested whether or not there was any relationship between perceived social support, contact with friends, contact with family, trust, participation, neighbourhood problems and ease of access to services and some health variables, after controlling for age and socio-economic measures. They found that [135]:

- Perceived severe lack of social support and trust in other people were significant predictors of poor self-assessed general health.
- Severe lack of social support was a strong predictor of a high GHQ12 score among both men and women and trust was also a predictor.
- Non-participation in organised activities was a strong predictor of cigarette smoking for both men and women.

The first two points are illustrated in Table 2.16.

Measuring social capital

There have been a large number of small-scale studies using a variety of instruments to capture different dimensions of social capital. In this section, we focus on the instruments used in the HSE in 2000, unless otherwise specified.

Measuring social networks

This includes:

- Perceived social support is measured through seven items about physical and emotional aspects of social support. This was originally

Table 2.16. *Impact of 'social capital' type variables*

	Men		*Women*	
Perceived social support	*Odds ratio*	*95% CI*	*Odds ratio*	*95% CI*
Odds of poor self-assessed health				
No lack of support	1.00		1.00	
Some lack of support	1.32	1.07–1.64	1.29	1.0–1.57
Severe lack of support	1.79	1.40–2.29	1.69	1.32–2.16
Odds of GHQ12 Scores of 4 or more				
No lack of support	1.00		1.00	
Some lack of support	1.58	1.20–2.09	1.41	0.94–1.39
Severe lack of support	2.97	2.23–3.97	3.35	2.59–4.33

Note: after controlling for age, social class of household reference person, household income, educational qualifications, car ownership and Townsend index of deprivation.

used in the Health and Lifestyle Survey [136], and has been used in HSE in 1994, 1995, 1998, 1999.

- Contact with family and friends is created from nine questions about whether informant had any contact with friends, family and neighbours in the previous fortnight.

Trust

The concept of trust was captured by three questions, taken from the General Social Survey in the U.S.:

- "Would you say that most of the time people try to be helpful or just look out for themselves?"
- "Do you think most people would take advantage of you if they got the chance or would try to be fair?"
- "Generally speaking, would you say that most people can be trusted or you cannot be too careful in dealing with people?"

Participation in organised activity

Measurement of social capital includes an estimate of participation in organised activity. This includes membership of groups and associations, including political groups, trade unions, environmental groups, parent/school associations, residents' groups or neighbourhood watch, participation in artistic, musical or educational activities through, for example, attending evening classes, religious groups including church attendance, groups for women, youth or the elderly, social or working men's clubs and sporting clubs. Problems can arise, because the pattern of participation in sporting activities is usually rather different from participation in other social activities.

Neighbourhood problems

Neighbourhood problems were measured through questions about: rubbish, graffiti and vandalism, teenagers hanging around, whether or not enjoying living with area, noisy neighbourhood/loud parties, not feeling safe walking alone after dark, problem of drunks/tramps, neighbours not looking after each other, and not having good local transport.

Ease of access to services

Questions to approximate access to services asked: How easy is it to get to a corner shop, a large supermarket, the post office, a general practitioner, an accident and emergency unit.

Summary and recommendations, and data sources

Although commonly used findings are ambiguous, so that it is unclear if these measures are adding a great deal to that explained by socio-demographic and socio-economic measures. However, if one is interested in using them, we would recommend scales that have been used by the national surveys.

SECTION 3

MEASURING INEQUALITY BY HEALTH AND DISEASE CATEGORIES (USING DATA FROM ADMINISTRATIVE SOURCES)

This section looks at how death and illness are recorded and measured by administrative data sources.

Administrative data used to identify health inequalities tend to be of one of two types:

- Mortality data (Section 3.1)
- Morbidity data from health service activity statistics, disease registers and similar official sources (Sections 3.2 and 3.3)

Two main types of data on health and disease are used to investigate inequalities:

- Data from administrative sources, including mortality data and health service activity data (Section 3).
- Data from surveys of health, based on samples from the general population or from people with particular conditions and/or receiving healthcare (Section 4).

3.1 Mortality Data

Mortality levels are expressed as incidence rates, calculated by:

$$\frac{\text{[observed number of deaths in the group, for specified period]}}{\text{[number of people in the group]} \times \left[\begin{array}{c}\text{average number of years of those}\\ \text{people alive for specified period}\end{array}\right]}$$

Using official data at a national, regional or local level, this usually implies dividing the number of deaths in a year by the national or regional population in the middle of that year (assuming that half of the deaths take place either side).

One-off studies that attempt to assess the death rates can be divided into longitudinal studies (where a cohort is followed up over a number of years) and cross-sectional studies.

- In longitudinal studies, the number of person years of exposure can be calculated directly from the data collected in the study.
- In unlinked cross-sectional studies, the denominator is usually estimated as the number of people in the middle year of the study period times the number of years covered by the study period.

Mortality rates for different groups

Different choices of groups and periods lead to a wide variety of mortality figures. Those commonly used are:

- The perinatal mortality rate.
- The infant mortality rate.
- The under 65 mortality rate.
- The 65 plus mortality rate.

Mortality data are commonly used to derive two other indicators: the standardised mortality ratio and the life expectancy.

Standardised mortality ratios (SMRs)

Comparison between different areas, groups or variations through time

Usually, one wants to compare the mortality level in one area with another, or of one group with another, or for the same group over time. In most cases, when assessing levels of inequality, one is focussing on comparisons between socio-economic strata.

The problem is that groups will differ in respects other than their socio-economic status. In particular, both age and sex are associated strongly with morbidity and, depending on the context, likely mortality. The usual practise, therefore, is to *standardise* for age and sex before making any comparison between socio-economic strata (Box 12).

Whilst using SMRs to make comparisons between groups or over time is standard practice, there are some caveats:

- Making and interpreting comparisons over time should be done with care, because the size of groups being compared change over time

Box 12

Standardisation

A standard set of mortality rates for age and sex groups are used and then applied to the age and sex composition of each of the groups under study. The common aim is to generate a predicted or expected number of deaths.

There are two main methods: the direct and indirect approach. The more common, indirect standardisation involves taking the national population figures and applying them to the age–sex breakdown in the local area to give an expected number. The observed number is then divided by the expected number to give the standardised value. Direct standardised death rates is the number of deaths that would be expected in the standard population if the age–sex specific death rates in the study population prevailed, divided by the size of the standard population.

The 'standardised ratio' is then calculated as the actual number of deaths divided by the expected number of deaths and conventionally multiplied by 100.

and the categories used to define the groups may change their meaning and significance. In particular, large variations between populations can give strange results [137].

- In the usual comparison of SMRs, the numbers of deaths involved is relatively small. This means that any change in the composition of the groups being compared can have a disproportionately large impact upon the relative SMRs, because those that move between groups may be more (or less) likely to die.
- Standardisation must be used thoughtfully because it may conceal important variations in the size of death or health inequalities according to age, sex, place of residence or other parameters that are used in the standardisation process.
- It may sometimes be better to present separate estimates for sub-groups of the population than to pool all differences in one standardised figure. For example, it is common to distinguish data for men and for women in nearly all measurements of health inequalities.
- Inskip [138] states that "standardised ratios can only be compared to the median of the distribution from which they are derived and not between two distributions". In other words, a standardised ratio is only standardised by reference to its parent distribution, for example, an SMR derived from Scottish data cannot be compared to an SMR derived from Welsh data.

- When used at a small area level, one should be aware of how small the numbers of deaths are.

SMRs are therefore not without problems. Moreover, in practice, the calculation of the SMR for each occupational social class at a given point in time involves comparison of the occupations as recorded at death with the occupational distribution at the most recent Census. Because the Census now appears to be better able to classify persons to more specific occupations than does the SMRs, there will be differences between the occupational distribution at the most recent Census and at the time of death (numerator–denominator bias) making SMRs unreliable for comparison over time.

In addition to the technical difficulties, anomalies and 'peculiarities' occur between different occupational social class classifications and the data do not always generate a clear gradient. Examples of specific problems include:

- Coding of social class at death may include important biases [139].
- Cause-specific mortality rates may be distorted by policy decisions about the relative importance of different disease categories using the International Classification of Diseases [139].
- Social stereotypes may affect coding of occupations, especially for those who have had a career of part-time or temporary jobs.

Box 13

Examples of 'peculiar' results found in analysis of these data sets include:

- The SMRs of commercial artists (occupation unit 020.21) is 107 whilst that of industrial designers (occupation unit 020.02) is 54.
- The SMRs of foremen responsible for product inspection and packing (occupational group 136) is 160 (based on 893 deaths) and that of industrial inspectors (occupation group 137) is only 71 (based on 3514 deaths).

Data sources

Small area mortality data are available from the ONS or from the Public Health Observatories. For further information contact the ONS helpdesk on the ONS website or www.apho.org.uk. The ONS published a paper on the options for small populations in 2003. Ward figures will be increasingly more available in the future.

Life expectancy

What does life expectancy mean?

Life expectancy at birth for an area in a particular period is an estimate of the number of years a new-born baby would survive, were he or she to experience the particular area's age-specific mortality rates for that time period throughout his or her life. The figure is calculated by applying those age-specific mortality rates to the progress of a hypothetical cohort of 100,000 year on year. Because the age-specific mortality rates are area and time specific, it reflects the current and previous conditions that have led people to die at different ages during that period.

It is important to emphasise that, life expectancy at birth is *not* the number of years a baby born in the area at that time could expect to live. This is because death rates of the area are likely to change in the future and because many of those born in the area will live elsewhere for at least some part of their lives.

Life expectancy can also be estimated at any age. It is sometimes denoted by a subscript, thus LE_{60} is the corresponding calculation for 60 year olds. There is no simple relationship between the life expectancies calculated for different ages. For example, if for a particular area, female life expectancy at birth is 80 years, it does not follow that life expectancy for someone aged 75 years is simply a further five years. This is because survival from a particular age depends on mortality rates beyond that age and the mortality rates for 75–79 years olds will have changed.

Proximity to death

Proximity to death is a recent addition to the lexicon of measures of health status.

Evidence shows that the bulk of healthcare expenditures for an individual is in the last few months of their life. There have even been suggestions that this should be the basis for resource allocation. However, it is difficult to see how this can be assessed prospectively, or how predictors of 'proximity to death' would outperform age distributions.

3.2 Morbidity Data from Health Service Activity Statistics, Disease Registers and Similar Official Sources

Other than Hospital Episode Statistics (HES), no comprehensive national small area health service activity data are collected in England. There are, however, a number of partial sources, though it may be difficult to negotiate access to data containing small area identifiers.

3.2.1 Summary of Data Sources

In this section, we describe the main sources available with brief notes on practical questions of access, availability and data quality.

These sources include:

- General Practice/Primary Care (Section 3.3.1)
  - General Practice Research Database.
  - Morbidity Statistics from General Practice (MSGP) publications.
  - Prescription Cost Analysis, Department of Health.
  - NHS Direct: triage database systems.
  - Regional Drug Misuse Databases.
  - Adult Dental Health Survey.
- Acute Sector (Section 3.3.2)
  - the Korner returns utilising Patient Administrative System (PAS) data from health authorities and trusts, comprising in-patient and outpatient data, for the HES.
- Community Health Sector (Section 3.3.3)
  - the Korner returns utilising PAS data.
- Disease Registers (Section 3.3.4).

3.3 General Practice/Primary Care Data

Previously, there was no central data archiving for general practice similar to that for hospital admissions and episode data. The history of general practice computing in England has not encouraged standardisation. The new GMS contract (nGMS) 2004 has lead to the availability of more information from primary care. The nGMS contract established the Quality Management and Analysis System (QMAS) which allows payment to be made to GPs under the Quality and Outcomes Framework (QOF).

<u>Local sources</u>

Small groups of practices have developed local patient databases for research, but there is no universal requirement for GPs to provide anonymised data on individual patients or consultations.

There are many examples of local projects successfully approaching general practices and primary care trusts for data on the incidence of specific problems or conditions. There may be no alternative to such local approaches if details on the severity of symptoms or clinical outcomes are required. The most promising conditions are those for which have standard care management protocols such as diabetes and asthma.

National sources

One officially supported data warehousing scheme has taken over the anonymised data collected by one of the main computer suppliers (VAMP) as part of its contractual arrangements with practices, whose original purpose was to assess drug safety through linking prescriptions to subsequent reports of side effects. This is known as the *General Practice Research Database (GPRD)* and is maintained by the Medicines and Healthcare Products Regulatory Agency for the Department of Health. It holds anonymised patient level data on reasons for consultation, diagnosis, prescribing and referrals. The number of contributing practices fluctuates, but in January 1999 there were 419 participating practices covering approximately three million patients. Their website says that "GPRD can be used to optimise decision-making across the health research spectrum including clinical epidemiology, drug safety, disease management and drug utilisation. It will be licensed to academics, regulators, pharmaceutical organisations and research service providers." Potential users should submit a request to the Scientific and Ethical Advisory Group: Medicines. More details can be found by contacting the Medicines' Control Agency.

The one comprehensive national resource on general practice activity covers *prescribing*. The *Prescription Pricing Authority (PPA)* keeps considerable detail on the prescribing behaviour of every English GP. Details include the volume/number of items of each drug prescribed and cost. Registered users have access to health authority level (and Primary Care Organization (PCO)) level data; anonymised GP or practice level data may be available to designated projects. These can be linked to data on the ward distribution of practice populations (as used in the past by health authorities for resource allocation) to generate small area maps of prescribing behaviour.

For several decades, the main national source of data on English General Practice have been the decennial surveys (carried out in 1955/1956, 1970/1971, 1981/1982 and 1991/1992) that have supported the series of *Morbidity Statistics from General Practice (MSGP)* publications. The MSGP4 was undertaken jointly by the ONS, the Royal College of General Practitioners and the Department of Health in 1991–1992. All general practitioners from 60 general practices recorded details of every face-to-face contact with their patients over the course of a year, and information on the socio-economic characteristics of all patients on their list was collected through a short interview questionnaire (Box 14). The total list size of the 60 practices was approximately 400,000. The sample of general practices is not representative in that only practices where all GPs agreed to participate in the study were used, and the practice had to collect certain information and use certain software which is not standard practice.

Box 14

Main topics covered by MSGP4:

Age, sex, socio-economic characteristics (region, urban/rural residence, housing tenure, marital status, household composition, social class, economic position, ethnic group), smoking status, number of consultations and referrals by ICD code, preventative healthcare, home visits, distance between patient's home and surgery.

The data are available as standard tables and data sets, customised tables and data sets, or as a package of data and analysis software from the ONS. For further information contact the ONS helpdesk.

The triage database systems used by *NHS Direct* are a potentially rich source of information on population morbidity, though it is not known to what extent the data includes a postcode or small area identifier. At present these data are periodically analysed in order to monitor presenting problems and referrals, but it is unclear to what extent the supporting data are publicly available. Please contact the NHS directly for more details.

Dental care is covered by Korner returns (Section 3.3.2), but these are unsuitable for small area analysis. Two decennial surveys are also available. The Adult Dental Health Survey (last conducted in 1998) involves interviews including a dental examination of approximately 5000 adults across the U.K. Because of the relatively small sample size, it is unlikely to generate reliable sub-regional results. A similar survey of children attending state schools in the U.K. generally has a sample exceeding 15,000. The most recent survey was conducted in 1993.

Other main sources of information on dental health are the claims submitted by dentists for NHS funded treatment. Information is published by HA on numbers and costs of courses of treatment, and more detailed data on types of treatment are extracted from a 5% sample of claims. It may be possible to access anonymised individual level data. The utility of these data will obviously depend on the local balance between NHS and private provision, which varies greatly across the U.K.

The *Regional Drug Users Databases* receive data from a number of sources, including local DAT teams, GPs, hospital trusts and support services. The aim is to keep an anonymised record of each contact between drug users and the support services. Results are collated centrally by the Department of Health and published in a biannual bulletin. The regional databases may be prepared to release anonymised data with ward level identifiers for local mapping exercises.

3.4 Acute Sector Data

The richest source of data, can be found in the *Korner* returns from health authorities and trusts. These cover almost all aspects of a trust's performance and include details of population morbidity as well as service activity and staffing levels. Returns are presented at trust or primary care trust level, and sometimes for units within trusts. Lower level data cannot be extracted from the central returns, though some of the contributing institutions may have compiled the material from systems that provide small area identifiers. High level summaries of Korner data are available on the Department of Health website.

The *Patient Administration Systems (PAS)* are one of several sources for the Korner returns. Several software suppliers produce PAS but they all have to comply with national standards for record structures. For in-patients, these include fields on length of stay, specialty and some diagnostic details. For outpatients, they will indicate the date of attendance, specialty and who was seen. Downloads from these systems are collated centrally to produce the familiar HES data. HES holds limited amount of clinical data – main and secondary diagnoses; it also contains age, gender, postcode and some details on referrals and outcomes. The data are available at a high level of aggregation from the ONS website.

Trying to retrieve more detailed clinical information from the acute sector can be very difficult. It will almost always require negotiation with individual trusts and, unless one is dealing with one of the minority of units that have computerised clinical records, it will involve extracting paper records from hospital archives.

3.5 Community Health Sector Data

The Community Health Sector is undergoing major re-structuring as community trusts are wound-down and responsibility for the majority of their services passes to PCOs. Prior to this re-structuring, data recording was very uneven. Although there are several PAS intended for community trusts, not all trusts used computerised systems; in the non-computerised trusts, the Korner returns are compiled manually.

Mental health trusts provide PAS returns for incorporation in HES data, but the quality of the data is thought to be patchy. There is likely to be some disruption to data recording where mental health trusts are forced to separate from combined community and mental health trusts. The National Programme for IT (NPfIT) aims to implement modern, integrated IT providing more efficient delivery of information.

SECTION 4

MEASURING INEQUALITY BY HEALTH AND DISEASE CATEGORIES (USING DATA FROM SURVEYS)

The purpose of this section is to show how health and disease can be measured through surveys and questionnaires.

For practitioners trying to decide whether to measure health inequalities in their region with a re-analysis of existing health data, this section offers guidance on the often bewildering quantity and variety of health, disease and 'lifestyle' surveys available, with some explanations on how these data have been acquired and caveats on their applicability and use.

For those wanting to collect new or different data, the section offers a guide to the range of different health and lifestyle questionnaires, the key types of health and disease measures used, the basic structure of questionnaires and surveys and their main strengths and limitations. (Section 9 provides a guide on how to carry out a survey).

The material is divided into three parts. The first (Sections 4.1 and 4.2) concentrates on the types of health and lifestyle surveys that are regularly employed in surveys of the general population.

The second part (Section 4.3) presents a selection of health status questionnaires that have (mainly) been developed for clinical and audit applications. The distinction between the sections is somewhat arbitrary as the shorter of the health status questionnaires are sometimes incorporated into health and lifestyle surveys, or even used as stand-alone instruments in epidemiological applications.

The third section provides a brief discussion on quality of life indexes.

4.1 Health and Lifestyle Surveys

4.1.1 What can be Covered by a Survey?

Most surveys of health and lifestyle aim to cover the topics listed in Table 4.1. Almost all of these topics were included in recommendations of the European 'Health for All' programme's contents of a questionnaire that could be used for cross-national monitoring of health and morbidity in Europe (Table 4.2). These topics are sufficiently well established. However, there is less agreement when it comes to choosing or devising measures for each topic; and the lack of standardisation makes for difficulties in comparing results.

The following sub-sections give more details of how health and lifestyle surveys tackle three of their main topic areas:

- Self-reported health and morbidity (Section 4.1.2).
- Physiological measurements (Section 4.1.3).
- Lifestyle and risk taking behaviours (Section 4.1.4).

4.1.2 Questions on Self-reported Health and Morbidity

Although self-reported health is often tackled by basic questions on how well (or ill) people feel, there are some more interesting and detailed efforts to get respondents to report recent symptoms. A common format is

Table 4.1. *Typical range of contents of a health and lifestyle survey*

Typical coverage of health in a large-scale health and lifestyle survey will include

Health, symptoms and disability:
- Perceived health
- Experience of illness and disease (based on checklist of symptoms and reports of any diagnosis supplied by medical professionals)
- Use of health and social care services
- A short battery such as the GHQ12, or parts of the Nottingham Health Profile to measure psychological malaise and well-being
- Reports of any disabilities, their presumed causes and impact on life
- Fitness

Examinations and physiological tests
- Some of the more ambitious surveys also employ nurses to carryout basic physiological tests, blood pressure, BMI and respiratory function.

Questions on lifestyle will at a minimum cover
- Diet
- Exercise
- Risk taking behaviour
- They may also include frequency and extent of social contacts, any caring roles, and support received.

Table 4.2. *Instruments for health interview surveys recommended for monitoring European Health For All indicators*

Health For All indicator (number)	*Health indicator general content*
Perceived health (2,2)	Percentage of respondents saying that their general state of health is very good, good, fair, poor or very poor.
Temporary disability (4,1)	Average number of days that respondents had to cut down their usual activities because of physical disability/mental conditions
Long-term disability (4,2)	A summary score derived from questions on confinement to bed, chair or house, difficulty in walking, dressing, washing, feeding, hearing, seeing, etc.
Prevalence of selected chronic conditions (4,6)	Physical health Mental health: batteries of questions on, respectively, dementia, mental retardation, and mental disorders
Emotional well-being	General health questionnaire: a summary score derived from questions on worry, concentration, feeling happy, etc.

Source: reproduced from Kunst and Mackenbach [7]. Previously adapted from third consultation to develop common methods and instruments for health interview surveys: report on a WHO meeting.

to present a list of symptoms (or conditions), proceeded by a question such as *"In the past month have you had any problems with . . .".* This model can be used in both interview and self-completion surveys (Table 4.3).

This method has certain difficulties:

- Lists of symptoms described in medical terminology may not be understood by everyone.
- The types of terms that are acceptable to a lay person may not be reliably translated into standard diagnoses or conditions.
- It does not capture the severity of symptoms.

The obvious alternative is to use open-ended questions that ask people to describe their symptoms and illnesses, but these are very difficult to code.

There have been attempts to validate the results of self-report check lists of symptoms against medical diagnoses and produce formulae for predicting most likely diagnoses from combinations of symptoms. Statistical techniques such as factor analysis have been used for this purpose, but it is unclear whether the results have any medical or epidemiological credibility.

Table 4.3. *Selections of common symptoms and problems typically used in self-completion surveys*

Column A	*Column B*
Topics for question of type: Have you had any trouble with x in past month	Possible list of conditions for self-report questionnaire
Headaches	Arthritis/rheumatism
Hay fever	Back trouble
Sleeping	Hernia
Constipation	Orthopaedic condition (excl back trouble)
Eyes	Heart disease, angina etc.
Bad back	High blood pressure
Nerves	Stroke, arterial disease
Colds and flu	Bronchitis, emphysema
Feet	Asthma
Tired	Respiratory TB
Kidney/bladder	Other respiratory disease
Joint pain	Stomach ulcer
Concentration	Other gastrointestinal diseases
Palpitations	Genitourinary diseases
Ears	Diabetes
Worry	Gout
Stomach	
Sinus	
Cough	
Faints	

The situation is very different for mental health questionnaires where this type of diagnosis-based validation is well established and the resulting instruments are employed for both screening and diagnosis.

4.1.3 Physiological Measurements and Surveys

If resources permit, researchers may try to incorporate a small set of physiological measurements in a survey. For example, interview-based surveys employ nurses to conduct physiological measurements on respondents:

- Levels of refusal can be quite high, and some surveys do not attempt to collect these data from older people (over 75 is a common cut-off point).
- Exercise can be both costly and difficult to arrange, especially when the measurements require technology that is not readily portable.
- Blood pressure and respiratory function are two measurements most often collected, but conventional interviews and self-completion methods can record details of height, weight and waist measurements.

- Height and weight are often used to generate a combined measure of physiological health in the form of the body mass index (BMI). BMI = weight (kg)/height $(m)^2$ (Table 4.4).

Table 4.4. *Recommended values for body mass index (BMI) Royal College of Physicians (RCP) (1983)*

	Males	*Females*
Underweight	20.0 and below	18.6 and below
Acceptable/normal	20.1–25.0	18.7–23.7
Mildly overweight	25.1–29.9	23.8–28.5
Obese	30.0 and above	28.6 and above

In theory, physiological measurements should not suffer from the problems of standardisation. However in practice, although the instruments themselves are technologically standardised, there is often disagreement on what are acceptable or problematic values. The guide values for BMI, one of the better established measures, are a case in point. In U.K., these are periodically reviewed and amended; internationally, different thresholds apply to different countries. What to take as critical threshold values for other indicators, such as volumetric flow measures for respiratory conditions, is the subject of much debate in the medical literature.

4.1.4 Surveys Measuring Health Behaviours (Lifestyle)

Although the usual outcome variable in a survey is a measure of ill health or morbidity, behaviour with respect to established risk factors to health are commonly employed in surveys. The usual focus is on the 'favourite four':

- Alcohol
- Diet
- Exercise
- Tobacco

Alcohol

Heavy alcohol consumption is associated not only with a higher risk of liver damage but also with heart disease, high blood pressure, cerebral vascular disease and other problems.

Alcohol consumption is measured in 'units', that correspond to standard amounts of pure alcohol in different alcoholic drinks. In principle, a unit corresponds to the amount of alcohol in a half-pint of ordinary strength beer or lager, a small glass of wine, or one measure of spirit. A person's weekly consumption of units is graded into 'Safe Drinking', 'Moderate Drinking' and

'Heavy Drinking'. This criteria has changed several times during the last twenty years.

The usual source of data is from a self-completion survey where respondents are asked to report on how many glasses of beer, lager, spirits and wine they have consumed during the last week. Clearly a person's self-assessment may be quite different from the above definition (e.g. what is 'ordinary' strength beer, how much is a glass?). In general, there is a tendency to under-estimate,[3] and the accuracy of both the recall and the assessment will vary between people.

Diet

In principle, measurement of a person's diet should include measurement of their intake of calories and protein and vitamins, etc., and consumption compared to standard values. This is an intensive and onerous data collection procedure (for both respondents and researchers) and is therefore usually only used for particular groups (e.g. young children).

In practice, therefore, except in specialised nutrition surveys, data collection and analysis are rarely that detailed. Instead, the more usual source of data is the self-report of the kinds and amounts of foods eaten during a fixed period. Comprehensive recording of foods consumed would also require an extensive data collection instrument, in which respondents would be asked to record whether or not they have consumed any one of a list of food items and how often during the reference period. Usual practice is to concentrate on 'marker' foods such as fruits, vegetables, bread and sugar.

There are all kinds of difficulties in interpreting survey responses because of variability in the quality and size of portions, as well as the usual problems of accuracy and recall. There are several ways for improving the usefulness of the data that is collected from surveys. For example:

- Respondents can be asked about their shopping habits and these data can be used to demonstrate inequalities in access to different kinds of food;
- Respondents can be asked about their cooking and eating habits.

Exercise

It is clear that some exercise is good for health, with considerable evidence linking lack of exercise to morbidity. However, apart from a physiological

[3] Thus, the national annual consumption estimated from national surveys of drinking behaviour is much lower than the volume estimated to have been sold based on customs and excise figures.

measure, units of energy expended, which is impractical to measure, there is no agreed standard set of measurements.

Some researchers use changes in pulse rate during exercise as a surrogate process measure, but this is also constrained to specific contexts such as in a gym. Others rely on self-reports of exercise taken during the previous week. The main difficulty lies in combining reports of different forms of exercise into a single measure.

Tobacco

Tobacco is associated not only with a higher risk of lung and other cancers, but also with heart disease, other cardio-vascular morbidity, and increased vulnerability to many other conditions.

Measurement should focus on nicotine intake but, of course, it is difficult to measure directly, especially when one wants to estimate levels of passive smoking.

The usual source of data is from a self-completion survey where respondents are asked to report on how many cigarettes or pipes of tobacco they have smoked during the last week. Although cigarettes (and cigars and tobacco) are clearly graded according to their nicotine content, there is no way of taking into account the extent to which smokers only smoke part of a cigarette. And, as with the above examples, there are the perennial problems of accuracy and of recall.

4.2 Regular Health and Lifestyle Surveys

Several surveys are routinely conducted to measure the health of the population of England. The major ones include:

- HSE (Box 15).
- Surveys of Psychiatric Morbidity in Great Britain.
- GHS.
- The Omnibus Survey.

HSE is a major tool for monitoring the nation's health. It has been conducted annually since the early 1990s and since 1995 the sample has included measurements of the heights of children aged 2–15 as well as adults. The survey consists of an interview and some basic physiological measurements. Every year the survey covers blood pressure, anthropometry, cigarette smoking, alcohol consumption and self-assessed general health. Each year there are also a set of special themes relating to particular aspects of physical functioning, symptoms and lifestyle. The data are available from the Data Archive at the University of Essex [140].

Box 15

The Health Survey for England

From 1991 to 1994, the survey focussed on cardiovascular disease and associated risk factors. In 1995 and 1996 the major focus of the survey was atopic disease (asthma, eczema, etc.), accidents and disability. In 1997, the survey report focussed on the health of young people aged 2–24, and combined data (in report only) from 1995–1997. In 1998, the focus was on cardiovascular disease. In 1999, the focus was on ethnic groups and in 2000, older people and social exclusion. In 2001 the focus was on non fatal accidents, disability, respiratory conditions, atopic conditions, fruit and vegetable consumption. In 2002 the focus was on the health of children and young people, the health of infants aged under one, and their mothers.

The Survey of Psychiatric Morbidity in Great Britain was conducted by Office for Population Censuses and Survey (OPCS) during 1993–1994. The survey was repeated in 2000. The report Psychiatric Morbidity Among Adults Living in Private Households, (2000) (is available from the ONS). It presents the findings of a survey of psychiatric morbidity among adults aged 16–74 living in private households in Great Britain that was carried out between March and September 2000. It was commissioned by the Department of Health, the Scottish Executive and the National Assembly for Wales. It is one of a series of surveys of different population groups which began in 1993 and is a repeat of the first of these surveys, which covered 10,000 adults aged 16–64 living in private households. The data for all these surveys is deposited at the Data Archive.

Both the GHS and the Omnibus Survey frequently have supplements relating to aspects of health and lifestyle.

GHS is a multi-purpose survey conducted by the Social Survey Division of the ONS. The survey started in 1971 and has been carried out continuously since then, except for a break in 1997–1998 and 1999–2000. The GHS is carried out for a number of government departments and provides information for planning and policy purposes, including to monitor progress towards achieving targets. Data are collected on housing, employment, education, health and family information from approximately 9000 households in Great Britain. The GHS has a modular structure and other subjects, e.g. elderly, smoking, drinking, contraception, hearing and childcare are covered periodically, and new topics are introduced from time to time. The data are available from the Data Archive at the University of Essex [140].

The Omnibus is a multi-purpose survey developed by ONS for use by non-profit organisations. The Omnibus allows customers to receive results quickly, yet retaining the hallmarks of high quality – a random probability sample, high response rates and advice on questionnaire design. The survey is carried out in two of the three months each quarter. Approximately 1800 adults are interviewed each survey month, and the average response rate is 65%.

Other health and lifestyle surveys

In addition to these, a variety of large-scale major health and lifestyle surveys have been conducted over the past twenty years, funded by commercial, charitable and government agencies at both national and sub-national levels. Their data still have considerable potential for reanalysis. The Data Archive holds the individual level data for many of these. Interview schedules for these surveys often exceed 50 pages in length. They frequently include short copyrighted health-status questionnaires such as the GHQ or parts of the SF-36.

4.3 Health Status and Symptom Report Questionnaires

4.3.1 Introduction

This section discusses a major growth area in health questionnaire development – the many hundreds of instruments (questionnaires and checklists) often intended for medical assessment, screening and outcomes measurement. Though some cover very similar themes to the health and lifestyle surveys, there is a difference of emphasis, as most of these are intended to provide a health score, or diagnostic assessment. Consequently, they may not be ideal for epidemiological purposes; they may have to be completed by a medical professional, and not be appropriate for use in interviews, and they may be too long for self-completion. Moreover, many are strongly copyrighted and can only be used with the author's or publisher's permission. This may be given freely when the purpose is to preserve the integrity of the instrument and ensure that a body of comparable data is developed. Some instruments can only be used on payment of licence fees. In both instances, it may be difficult to obtain details of the scoring systems of the instruments without approaching the authors or publishers.

Fortunately, there are several detailed and wide-ranging reviews that can assist in the selection of a suitable measure [5,141,142]. Ann Bowling has produced some of the most comprehensive reviews in this area *Measuring Health* [4] and *Measuring Disease* [143] give details and references for several hundred of the more widely used measures.

Instruments tend to cluster into two overlapping groups. The first is the *generic model* which seeks to establish standard universal measurements of health that can be applied to any group in any setting. The interest in standardisation may arise from a simple concern to minimise confusion and duplication of effort, or, it may be part of a drive to establish common databases for the monitoring and planning of healthcare (Box 16).

Box 16

Gold Standard for the Measurement of Health

"To meet the needs of the 1990s, information about general health outcomes must be added to the nation's healthcare database. Minimum standards of comprehensiveness should be adopted to monitor the health of the general population and evaluate healthcare policies. A core set of generic health outcome measures should be standardised and adopted to compare the relative burden of medical and psychiatric conditions and relative treatment benefits. It is now practical to include a standardised core set of general health measures across applications (e.g. general population surveys, clinical trials) while supplementing this core according to the needs of a given study. The resulting comparisons would greatly advance understanding of the interpretation of health measures for all applications. Adoption of a standardised core set of health measures should be a high priority" (Source: *SF-36 Manual*, ch. 11 p.18).

This approach assumes there are universal constructs of physical, mental and social health across similar cultures and societies. If an instrument is a valid measure of these constructs then measurements can be compared between different settings and between groups with different medical conditions.

Most Multi-dimensional Health Status Profiles (MDPs) and indices, such as quality of life years lost, are grounded in this generic approach.

The second direction of development for health status measures could be described as the *condition specific model*. Unlike the generic approach it is not concerned to establish global standards and may question the validity of such standards. Rather, it aims to develop instruments that reflect the priorities and perspectives of groups with particular conditions, or those who are in receipt of similar kinds of healthcare. Some of these instruments will cover specialised topics, others measure more general health status. But the choice of domains, the associated definitions and selection of items, take account of specific interests.

The two approaches differ on their preferred strategies for developing and testing instruments. Evidence on the properties of the instruments, such as correlations with other measures, and demographic variations in

Table 4.5. *Advantages and limitations of generic measures*

Advantages of generic measures

- More likely to have been extensively developed
- Psychometric properties may be better known
- More likely to have supporting baseline/normative data from population and patient surveys
- Constructs may be sufficiently general to be widely relevant
- Provide an overview of health status/impact of illness from a single instrument
- Relatively cost-effective approach, provided the domains are independent and relevant

Limitations

- Can be hard to tell precisely what they mean and measure; this can present difficulties when selecting instruments and interpreting results
- May miss critical factors for individual conditions, interventions or patient groups
- May collect superfluous data; only a subset of domains are relevant to most applications
- May be oversensitive to effects of confounding factors
- May not provide sufficiently specific information for a number of administrative and audit applications such as: evaluating quality of care, monitoring variations in protocols and interventions, or planning the details of service development

scores, may be interpreted differently. The generic model may place more emphasis on psychometric criteria in the testing and developing of measures (Table 4.5), while the condition-specific model approach may stress qualitative methods of testing for validity and acceptability, alongside psychometric criteria.

The instruments

This section briefly introduces some of the major instruments under the following headings, indicating which are most likely to be suitable for use in surveys:

4.3.2 Measures concentrating on physical symptoms, functioning and general health.
4.3.3 Measures of mental health and mental illness.
4.3.4 Measures of social adjustment.
4.3.5 Measures of social support.
4.3.6 Measures of children's health.
4.3.7 Measures for older people.
4.3.8 Measures for people with specific conditions:
- cancer.
- asthma and respiratory conditions.

4.3.9 Multi-dimensional Health Profiles (MDPs).
4.3.10 The Health Index.

This is only a selection of the available instruments, which have been selected because, in our view, are the most likely to be suitable for measuring health inequalities. The criteria used to make the selection include the following:

- Brevity (number of items)/time and ease of administration questionnaires it should be suitable for postal use.
- Suitable for use by non-specialist interviewers.
- Wording and topic coverage that is suitable for self-completion (e.g. they should not induce anxiety or distress).
- Availability of published results – though this could range from one specialised study to a large body of publications with supporting databases of results from prior studies.
- Some evidence of psychometric properties and other tests of validity.

Not all of our selections meet all these criteria. When possible, we will note major drawbacks, but our knowledge is limited to only a sample of the literature on most of these instruments. Moreover, there are simply not enough publications on a number of the measures to be able to make all these judgements.

For more detail, we strongly recommend the two books by Ann Bowling (Section 4.3.1). Coverage of instruments produced post-2000 may be patchy.

Finally, we must emphasise that the following should be treated as a list of suggestions rather than recommendations.

4.3.2 Measures Concentrating on Physical Symptoms and Functioning

Functional status measures

These are some of the oldest heath status questionnaires and are designed to monitor levels of disability as they affect the performance of basic activities such as feeding, dressing and bathing. They are also known as indexes of Activities of Daily Living (ADL), or as measures of dependency. They have been mainly developed for use in institutional settings and are often intended for rapid assessments by health professionals. More recent versions cover tasks more associated with living in the community, such as shopping and cooking.

Two of the best known in this group – the Barthel Index [144] and the WHO Functional Scale (WHO, 1979) – are only suitable for use by medical professionals. However, both are quick and relatively easy to complete, and provide simple overall assessments (e.g., the WHO instrument rates people on a 5-point scale). They, or similar measures of dependency, could be included in standard electronic records for older people needing nursing or residential care, or high levels of domiciliary care. The Royal College of Physicians and The Royal College of General Practitioners have recommended the Barthel Index for screening elderly people in general practice.

Several instruments exist in multiple versions – some intended for professional assessment and some for self-completion. It is worth considering a self-completion version of the Functional Status Index [145]. This is predominately intended for use with adults suffering from arthritis, but even the short 18-item version covers the full range of topics associated with an ADL measure.

There are several questionnaires to assess functional status in the general population that have epidemiological potential. The Sickness Impact Profile (SIP) [146], though originally intended to measure changes in behaviour due to sickness and the outcomes of care, has been suggested for use in health surveys, though the full 136-item schedule is too long for self-completion. The Functional Limitations Profile (FLP) [147] is a modified version of SIP intended for use in the U.K. rather than the United States. Patrick et al. [148] have also developed the Lambeth Disability Screening Questionnaire, a checklist which is available in two versions; one for households, including questions such as: "does anyone in the household have difficulty with. . .?", and another for individuals. Both are intended to be used to identify levels of disability in a population, as well as a screening instrument to identify individuals or households with problems.

Currently, functional status is as likely to be measured by a domain taken from a multi-dimensional instrument, than a single topic measure. The Medical Outcomes Survey (MOS) instruments (of which the SF-36 is the best known) have sections on functional status which are discussed later. The Multi-dimensional Functional Assessment Questionnaire (MFAQ) – developed for the Older Americans Resources and Services Program (Duke University paper 1972–1975) – is a multi-dimensional health measure, but its first section (intended for interview) is a wide ranging checklist for assessing function in older people.

Many condition-specific instruments have short sections on functional status that could be employed in population surveys, especially with older people. One of the most relevant is the Stanford Health Assessment Questionnaire (HAQ), [149], originally intended for use with adults suffering from arthritis, but equally useful as a short general assessment of the difficulty of performing everyday tasks.

Measures of pain

A wide range of instruments are available both for measuring pain in general and pain associated with specific, often chronic, conditions.

Several measures concentrate on pain associated with musculoskeletal disorders. A few of the better known examples include the Back Pain

Classification Scale [150]; sections of the Arthritis Impact Measuring Scale (AIMS2) [151]; and the Oswestry Low Back Pain Disability Questionnaire.

More general coverage is provided by the lengthy McGill Pain Questionnaire, while the Self-rating Pain and Distress Scale [152] is intended as a brief measurement of mood and behaviour changes associated with acute pain.

Several of the MDPs (Section 4.3.9) contain items referring to pain. These include all versions of the MOS questionnaires, from the 149-item version to the SF-6, the Dartmouth Coop Function Charts and the Nottingham Health Profile.

4.3.3 Measures of Mental Health and Mental Illness

There are many measures of mental health and illness, mostly concerning depression. They are often well established, widely validated and theoretically based.

There are several groups of measures. One set is concerned with cognitive functioning, especially in older people, and include tests of memory and general knowledge. The 10-item Mental Status Questionnaire [153] has been widely used and has been influential in the development of subsequent instruments such as the Comprehensive Assessment and Referral Evaluation Schedule CARE [154]. Even in its short form, CARE is probably too long for survey use; it is also rather specialised, with a focus on distinguishing dementia from depression in the elderly. However, there are several shorter instruments intended to establish the incidence of memory problems and the onset of dementia that might be practical for surveys. These include the community version of the Geriatric Mental State Test [155] and various versions of the Mental Status Questionnaire [156–159]. The Hodgkinson abbreviated Mental Test Score and Mental Test [160] are two further short tests of memory and confusion.

There are several widely used screening instruments for depression whose shorter forms appear quite regularly in population health surveys. The Carroll Rating Scale for Depression [161] is a self-administered version of the Hamilton Rating Scale for Depression [162]. Better known are the General Health Questionnaire [163], which, despite its title, is a measure of psychiatric symptoms, predominately depression, the Beck Depression Inventory [164] and the Zung Self-rating Depression Scale [165]. Anyone planning to use extracts from these instruments in surveys should note that permission may be required to reproduce the questions.

Slightly more general measures of mental health in the community have been produced. The 38-item Mental Health Inventory [166] (developed as part of the MOS programme) is the longest of these. It has been used in several large surveys to measure psychological distress and well being. However, unless one is intending to dedicate an entire survey to mental health issues, it may be preferable to use shorter mental health assessments, such as the section on mental health in the SF-36. Most Multi-dimensional Profiles include short sections on mental health.

4.3.4 Measures of Social Adjustment

Measures of social adjustment are closely related to measures of mental health. They attempt to record the extent of 'feeling at home' in the local community and the ability to cope with immediate social surroundings. They are frequently, but not exclusively, intended for use with older people, but other measures (or parts of longer measures) are concerned with the problems of social activity and integration for people with severe physical conditions.

A few instruments are designed exclusively to measure social adjustment. The Katz Adjustment Scales [167] concentrate on the social adjustment of psychiatric patients following treatment, but parts of it could be more widely used. The Crichton Royal Behaviour Scale is intended for use in residential care and requires an assessor who knows the person being assessed. Again, most of the longer measures of health status include sections on social adjustment, which could be extracted (with permission) for specific applications. For most purposes, it may be helpful to combine such an extract on social adjustment with a measure of social activity or social support.

4.3.5 Measures of Social Support

While measures of social adjustment record an individual's perceptions of their surroundings, measures of social support focus on the links between the individual, their family and the community. They measure the level and quality of contact with friends and relatives. Predictably, they can be very culturally specific, including questions on memberships of community organisations such as clubs, societies and churches that are unlikely to be relevant to all groups of respondents. The HSE has contained a standard set of items on social support since 2000.

4.3.6 Children's Health

There is a well-established tradition of various forms of mental health, intelligence and psychiatric screening tests for children. There are also a few instruments recording the symptoms of children with specific conditions, especially childhood cancers [168] and asthma [169,170]. However, there are very few measures for children and most are completed by proxy.

Bowling in 1997 [4], noting the lack of measures for children, comments that "there have been attempts to develop scales for children . . . , but these are (still) relatively under-used". She goes on that "Medical Outcomes Trust in the U.S., together with the Children's Health and Quality of Life Project team have recently developed child health forms for age groups 5–15 and infant pre-school, which are parent completed, and middle childhood–adolescent, which are completed by the child" [171].

4.3.7 Measures for Older People

Most of the functional status measures and Instrumental Activities of Daily Living (IADL), covering more social topics than ADL scales, are predominately intended for use with older people, though not necessarily validated. Indeed, many of the older functional status measures are better regarded as measures of dependency, or the need for nursing support, rather than measures of general health or health concerns.

Widely used examples of questionnaires covering the impact of health and disease on the life of older people include the already mentioned FLP and the Lambeth Disability Screening Questionnaire (Section 4.3.2), whose 25 items cover mobility both at home and outside, specific physical functions and impact on daily activities. The 22 items of the individual version cover a similar range of topics. Both versions may be distributed by post for self-completion or may be used in interviews.

The MFAQ (Section 4.3.2) could be regarded as a general MDP, but as already noted, its first section which is intended for interview, is an extensive checklist for assessing function in older people.

Some of the MDPs (including the SF-36) are criticised for focussing too heavily on relatively high levels of physical mobility and activity, such as sports performance, and fail to cover the sorts of everyday tasks, that may be problematic for older people. It is important not to assume that general health status questionnaires will validly represent the health status of older people. This is an area in which it is particularly important to pilot an instrument before use.

Several of the instruments mentioned earlier, under 'mental health', were designed to distinguish dementia from depression in older people. These include the community version of the Geriatric Mental State Test [155] and several versions of the Mental Status Questionnaire [156–159]. The Hodgkinson abbreviated Mental Test Score and Mental Test [160] are the two further short tests of memory and confusion that are mainly administered to older people.

4.3.8 Questionnaires for People with Specific Conditions

There are questionnaires to record symptoms, and experiences of coping with both treatment and symptoms, for most major medical conditions. By their very nature they are unlikely to be suited to general population use. However, a population survey might want to include questions on the symptoms of some of the more widespread conditions such as asthma. These instruments may help map inequalities in the outcomes of care, symptom management and impact on life.

Caution is required, as most of these instruments are usually administered in controlled settings, often as part of a care regime. Although most are sufficiently short and clear to be used in wider surveys, it is unclear whether they are ideal or appropriate for this purpose. It may also be unethical to use some of the instruments relating to cancer and mental health, without providing respondents with counselling or some form of support.

Measures for people with cancer

There are many questionnaires to monitor the health status of people with cancer, most of which include items on the side-effects of interventions. They have a long history; the Karnofsky Performance Status Scale, a very limited assessment of ability to perform normal activities, was published in 1949.

Some of the shorter instruments include:

- The European Organisation for Research on Treatment of Cancer (EORTC) has developed core questionnaires with 30 and 36 items and various modules relevant to specific cancers [172–174].
- The Rotterdam Symptom Checklist has been recommended by an MRC working party and exists in various forms mostly with 30–40 items [175].
- Fayer and Jones produced a diary card for cancer sufferers that is sometimes referred to as the Medical Research Council Scale, which records details of vomiting, activity, mood, anxiety and overall health [176].

It is not always clear whether such measures are intended to test for side-effects of therapies in clinical trials, or to monitor and treat in individual patient care.

Some of the more widely used short instruments for self-completion (or interview) include:

- The Cancer Functional Living Index [177];
- The short version of the Cancer Rehabilitation Evaluation System (CARES) [178].
- The Ontario Cancer Institute/Royal Marsden Scale [179].
- The Cancer Quality of Life Index [180,181].

Measures for people with asthma and respiratory conditions

At least 10 major instruments have been developed for measuring health status and quality of life of asthmatics in clinical trials. Most of these are too long and elaborate to use in routine care or population surveys.

For example, two of the more patient-centred instruments are the Living With Asthma Questionnaire [182] and the Asthma Quality of Life

Questionnaire [183]. Both were developed from interviews and group work with patients.

In the group work to develop the first of these, Hyland's participants reported effects of their condition that could be grouped under 11 headings: social/leisure, sport, holidays, work and other activities, sleep, colds, mobility, use of medications, effects on others, comments on doctors, dysphoric states and attitudes to asthma. Physical symptoms were excluded from the final 68-item questionnaire, as the aim was to develop an instrument that concentrated on disability.

Asthmatics who participated in Marks' groups were asked to consider the impact of their asthma on most aspects of their life, including: usual functioning, moods, feelings and relationships, and the consequent restrictions on life and overall well being. Though they were not asked about physical symptoms, these were mentioned spontaneously in discussion. Participants mentioned: physical symptoms, physical incapacity, control issues, emotional states, role fulfilment, social interaction and general health perceptions. Based on the suggestions, principal component analysis suggested six core domains: breathlessness (shortness of breath and reports of physical activities that induced breathlessness), concerns (mainly general concerns for health and future, but also feelings of lack of control and dependency on medication), control (understanding, feelings of coping and being in control), cough (sputum, congestion and cough), mood (a combination of fatigue and anxiety), social (restrictions on social life and sport, feelings of underachievement).These are all covered in the resulting 20-item questionnaire.

Shorter versions are being developed. Though too long for regular use in routine care, these instruments give an indication of the full range of outcomes that might be considered, the interrelation between the different outcomes, and an idea of what is most important to patients. They are typical of instruments designed to be administered to people with specific medical conditions.

4.3.9 Multi-Dimensional Health Status Profiles

MDPs represent a relatively recent approach to health status measurement. They cover several dimensions of health that might have previously been measured with separate instruments. (Box 17).

MDPs range in length from more than 140 to less than 10 questions and all but the shortest provide information on at least six different dimensions of illness and health. There are between 10 and 20 of these instruments in reasonably common use and most of these major instruments are listed in Table 4.6. As far as length/cost of administration/completion time is concerned, they can be considered in three groups: those with less than 15 questions (normally used alongside other instruments); those with 15–50 questions; and those with more than 50 items.

Box 17

A multi-dimensional picture of an individual's health

It takes 5–10 min to complete the 36 items on the SF-36 questionnaire, and there are several scoring schemes that provide a health profile such as the following based on the instrument's nine domains.

Physical functioning	95%
Social functioning	70%
Energy/vitality	40%
Physical impact on social role	80%
Emotional impact on social role	60%
Mental health	65%
Experienced pain	80%
General health	65%

It is typical of the sort of picture provided by an MDP questionnaire.

MDPs are *profiles* (Sections 7.2 and 7.4.3) in that they separately report results for each of their constituent domains. Many oppose attempts to collapse these scores to a single number and turn the profile into an index, but there is a great deal of interest in ways of doing this. Much of this comes from healthcare purchasers, planners, administrators, policy makers and associated researchers. They require an index with a single score for overall health that can be used for purposes such as comparing the health gain produced by different services, units and interventions. In one respect,

Table 4.6. *Some of the more widely used multi-dimensional health profiles*

Name of instrument	*Number of items*	*Number of scored dimensions*
Duke–UNC Health Profile	63	4
Duke Health Profile (17-item selection from Duke–UNC Profile)	17	4 (6)
Nottingham Health Profile Ptl	38	6
Sickness Impact Profile and Functional Limitations Profile (U.K. version of SIP)	136	12 (2)
Dartmouth Co-op Function Charts	9	9
McMaster Health Index Questionnaire	68	3
Medical Outcomes Survey (MOS) Full 149-item Functioning and Well-Being Profile (FWBP)	149	35 (8)
MOS FWBP-C (condensed version of full instrument)	113	20 (4)
MOS short form – 36-item instrument	36	9
MOS short form – 20-item instrument	20	6
MOS short form – 6-item instrument	6	6
EuroQol (6-item profile)	6	6

indexes and profiles are not radically different, as most profiles use the principles of indexation to combine component/item scores within each domain. Nevertheless, this type of indexation seems more widely acceptable than collapsing the different domains into a single number, partially because the single value index assumes that the same weightings for different aspects of health will be valid for all groups of respondents.

Domain coverage

Most MDPs cover a similar range of core topics, though they may describe them rather differently. The domain names of several MDPs are listed in Table 4.7. Domains with similar names may be measured in quite different ways, with different sets of components and different abilities to measure change or record extreme values. It is common to find them containing items that are culturally specific, or more appropriate to people of certain ages or health status. Table 4.7 lists the domain coverage of the main instruments, but, copyright permitting, it may be best to mix and match sections from different instruments. When doing so, it is worth remembering that factor analysis or related statistical techniques may have been used to maximise the independence of domains and that sections from several instruments are unlikely to have the same degree of independence. However, this is unlikely to pose serious problems unless the domain scores are to be combined into an overall rating of health.

It is worth considering using MDPs when:

- There is a need for self-reports of health and the impact of illness in non-clinical terms.
- These need to cover a relatively standard range of topics.
- There is a need to supplement conventional bio-medical assessments.
- There is a need for 'generic' measures to produce information for comparing different services and interventions.

MDPs may not be useful when:

- Resources are very limited and very specific information is required.
- Data of immediate relevance to services are required for audit and assessment.
- There is a need for a single index value of health.

Most self-report multi-dimensional instruments are likely to be more sensitive to non-health service influences than more specific or clinical measures, so it can be difficult to decide what part of any effects are due to health services or their lack.

The relationship between what these instruments measure and lay perceptions of health and health concerns are rarely clear. Before

Table 4.7. *Domain coverage of some major MDPs*

Name of instrument	*Number of items*	*Methods of application*	*Scored dimensions*	*Number of scored dimensions*
Duke–UNC Health Profile	63	I S	Symptom status, physical function, emotional function, social function	4
Duke Health Profile (17-item selection from Duke–UNC Profile)	17	S	Physical health, social health, mental health, general health	4 (6)
Nottingham Health Profile Ptl	38	I S	Physical mobility, pain, sleep, energy, social isolation, emotional reactions	6
Sickness Impact Profile and Functional Limitations Profile	136	I I A S	Categories: ambulation, body care and movement, mobility, household care and management, recreation and pastimes, social interaction, emotion, alertness, sleep and rest, eating, communication. Dimensions: physical, psychosocial	12 (2)
Dartmouth Co-op Function Charts	9	I A S	Physical condition, emotional condition, daily work, social activities, pain, change in condition, overall condition, social support, quality of life	9
McMaster Health Index Questionnaire	68	I T S	Physical functions (physical activities, mobility, self-care, communication); emotional functions (self-esteem, personal relationships, critical life events, thought about the future); social functions (general well-being, work, social role performance, material welfare, family participation and friendships)	3

Table 4.7. *(Continued)*

Name of instrument	*Number of items*	*Methods of application*	*Scored dimensions*	*Number of scored dimensions*
Medical Outcomes Survey (MOS) full 149-item Functioning and Well-Being Profile (FWBP)	149		Physical functioning, satisfaction with physical ability, mobility, role limitations due to physical health, role limitations due to emotional problems, unable to work due to health, unable to do housework due to health, social activity limitations due to health, sexual problems, satisfaction with family life, overall happiness with family life, marital functioning, anxiety (I and II), depression/behavioural emotional control (I and II), positive affect (I and II), feelings of belonging, cognitive functioning, current health, prior health, health outlook, health concern, resistance to illness, health distress, energy/fatigue, sleep quantity, optimal sleep, sleep disturbance, sleep adequacy, sleep somnolence, sleep shortness of breath or headache, snoring	35 (8)
MOS FWBP-C (condensed version of full instrument)	113		20 scales and 4 summary indexes	20 (4)
MOS Short form – 36-item instrument	36		Physical functioning, role functioning/physical, role functioning/emotional, energy/fatigue, emotional well-being, social functioning, pain, general health, health change	9
MOS Short form – 20-item instrument	20		Physical functioning, role functioning, social functioning, mental health, health perceptions, pain	6
MOS Short form – 6-item instrument	6		Physical functioning, role functioning, social functioning, psychological distress/well-being, health perceptions, pain	6

considering their use in population surveys it is important to test whether the items accurately reflect the concerns of major users of healthcare, such as older people. The utility of a general questionnaire may be diminished if the phenomena of interest tend to be concentrated in large sub-groups of the population, for which a general instrument may not be well suited.

Most MDPs have been subjected to basic psychometric assessments, both during their development and subsequently. The testing tends to concentrate on the capacity to measure change over time (as required for use in clinical trials), but it may have some relevance to epidemiological applications. More details of the tests can be found in Section 7.

4.3.10 A Single Health Rating – the Health Index

Several of the MDPs described above provide scoring systems to aggregate the separate domain scores into an overall health rating. The approach is very attractive to policy makers because it provides a single measure on which to evaluate the gains that can be achieved by healthcare interventions and hence to devise standards for cost effectiveness. The difficulty is how to translate the overall health rating into a metric that can be compared with the resource inputs of different interventions. We consider two approaches: Disability Adjusted Life Expectancy (DALE) and Quality Adjusted Life Years (QALYs).

Disability Adjusted Life Expectancy

Measures of life expectancy can be adjusted to take account of disability, hence DALE or DALYs.

Measures that adjust life expectancy for disability have been used since the beginning of the 1970s when both Japan and the U.S. presented data on Life Expectancies Adjusted for Disability (LEADS). The Japanese calculations illustrated the effect of various adjustments (Table 4.8).

Table 4.8. *Average life expectancy and average loss of years due to health impairments*

Age	*Year*	*Average life expectancy (a)*	*Loss due to illness (b)*	*Losses due to mental or physical disabilities (c)*	*Average loss (b + c − overlap) (d)*	*Average life expectancy minus average loss (a–d)*
0	1966	70.88	2.00	0.94	2.80	68.08
	1970	71.93	2.35	0.98	3.15	68.78
15	1966	57.38	1.83	0.90	2.59	55.20
	1970	58.45	2.13	0.91	2.89	55.56
65	1966	13.81	0.78	0.47	1.18	12.63
	1970	13.97	0.91	0.51	1.35	12.62

The adjustments attenuated improvements (compare columns (*a*) and (*d*)), but the differences were obviously small. It is interesting to note that at the time, the LEADS were abandoned as an overall measure of health status.

With increasing longevity, these measures have become more widely used, and the OPCS has produced a manual on how these are calculated and how to interpret them [184].

These measures are similar to the DALYs used by the World Bank as a tool for prioritising and targeting healthcare interventions in many developing countries. The problem for using such an approach is that relying only on disabilities as a measure of ill health is relatively restricted, and health means different things to different people. Moreover, the logic of the measures has been criticised by Williams [185] as not taking into account the possible effectiveness of interventions; he and other economists have therefore searched for a method that explicitly focuses on the possible outcomes of healthcare interventions.

Quality adjusted life years

Their approach is to base the algorithm for converting the overall health rating into a metric on people's preferences for different states of (ill)health. They have conducted surveys where people evaluate different states of (ill)health. Various methods – for example, time trade-off in which people are asked to compare the value of being in state A for *n*(a) years compared to state B for *n*(b) years are used to convert these evaluations into a 'Q' or quality value, that is constrained to be between 0 (worst health) and 1 (best health). These 'Q's are used for weighting or 'adjusting' the years during which people are in those states of (ill) health, and the assessment of the cost effectiveness is then made by comparing the number of QALYs that are saved through the intervention.

This approach raises a number of problems. First, health means different things to different people (Box 18). Even in the very first study of this kind, doctors and patients had different views [186]. The QALY procedure is supposed to be 'democratic' because people are asked to rate health status. In fact, they are constrained by the design of the questionnaire instruments [187].

Box 18

Health means different things to different people

For example, Blaxter [188] identifies four dimensions of health:

- Unfitness or fitness.
- Disease and impairment or their absence.
- Experienced illness or freedom from illness.
- Psycho-social malaise or well being.

In addition, should we value patients or groups of patients equally, the QALY gives decreasing weights to older people (because they have lower life expectancies) and, therefore, less years that can be gained or saved through the intervention. However, there is survey evidence that the young and old alike place more weight on parents with young children and less on the old and very young [189].

People who suffer from illness generally adapt; and even if they do not adapt, their perceptions change. Some people may be more independent than others; in particular, older people, when asked, will still claim to be satisfied with their health [189] even though 'objectively' health deteriorates with age. This is because of the way in which the index is constructed by giving a 'floor' of 0 that most (although not all) interpret as equivalent to death, which means that the quality scores tend to be compressed towards one (the 'ceiling').

The final value of the QALY is calculated by adding together the years of life left and each year being weighted by '*Q*' and then discounted on the basis that future years are worth less then current years. Typically, a 3% discount rate is used. There is little survey evidence to support this. High discount rates lead to a bias against educational or other interventions at young ages.

Planning context

Given the move towards public participation, is it appropriate to introduce an index as a basis for decision making where only a limited number of 'experts' are conversant with the criticisms?[4] The costs per QALY or cost per DALY figures are based on average costs. Such figures are sub-optimal, and may not be easily transferred from one context to another (let alone from one country to another). Marginal costs of an additional intervention may be different from average costs. Given the other problems of interpretation, the public may well prefer disaggregated figures to overall DALY or QALY results.

[4] Of course, one cannot expect everyone to be conversant with the statistical calculations and technical procedures underlying many such indexes; but we are referring here to the issues of valuation (discussed under the theoretical heading above).

SECTION 5

AN INTRODUCTION TO THE USE OF INDEXES TO MEASURE DEPRIVATION

5.1 Background

Although there is not a great deal of consensus on the meaning of deprivation, there is rather more agreement that it is a multi-dimensional phenomenon. Two problems ensue:

- The measurement problem: how to represent these different dimensions with a single measure.
- The problem of data availability: are there sufficient data sources for all the key dimensions.

Both problems are covered by this section, together with methods for evaluating indexes. This section focuses on measuring deprivation, Section 7 gives a more general description of the structure and testing of indexes. More details of the indexes themselves are provided in Section 6.

5.1.1 Measuring a Multi-dimensional Phenomenon

An *index* of deprivation will typically have several *domains* (or dimensions) covering topics such as income, health and housing. Within each of these domains there may be several *indicators* (or components), such as different types of claimant counts in the income domain. These indicators are combined, often by weighted addition, to produce domain scores; then the domain scores are summed to give an overall index score. The values of the weights are critical as they control the contribution each indicator makes to the overall score. There are various statistical methods for both determining the weights and for selecting suitable indicators, but such choices are often made by researchers and policy advisors without recourse to statistics. More details can be found in Sections 7 and 10.3.

Depending on the context, it may be desirable to present the domain scores as well as the overall scores, thus preserving an element of multi-dimensionality. Traditional indexes of deprivation mainly provide a single score, but separate domain scores are published for more recent indexes such as the Index of Multiple Deprivation-2000 and 2004.

5.1.2 Presenting the Results from an Index

Results from indexes are presented in many different ways. The options are discussed in more detail in Section 10, but here are some of the main possibilities:

Raw scores. To say that an electoral ward has a score of −25 on the Jarman Index is fairly meaningless, though the use of raw scores may be appropriate if the values are to be used in some sort of statistical analysis or modelling.

Percentiles and probabilities are more commonly used than raw scores. These results are often concerned with whether the score for a particular area lies within, say, the 10% highest or lowest groups. When making this type of judgement it is helpful if the index produces scores with a known statistical distribution as this can be used to estimate the probability of being in a certain range.

Rankings are a popular form of presentation. Areas are ranked to reach conclusions on, for example, what are the 10% most deprived areas. For this, one needs to know nothing of the overall distribution of all potential scores on the measure.

Abstract or interpreted? For most indexes the values have no direct or simple meaning, and differences between values cannot be given substantive interpretation. We cannot say that one area is twice as deprived as another because one has double the deprivation score of the other. There are a few exceptions when, because of their method of derivation, the values of an index can be directly interpreted. For example, the index described by Gordon and Forrest [190] are predictions of the proportion of people in a locality who meet the Breadline Britain criterion of poverty. The disadvantage with such interpretations is that they may be misleading and without periodic revalidation, one cannot be sure that they will remain correct over time.

5.1.3 What to Put in an Indicator of Deprivation

To understand what comprises an indicator of deprivation, one needs to address three basic questions:

- What is the nature of deprivation? Is it a state of 'want' – a predominantly 'natural' condition; or the result of a process in which something is withheld, or wherein people are excluded.
- What is the 'content' of deprivation, what do people lack, from what are they excluded, or what is being withheld? Classically, this is some form of income or wealth, but most contemporary approaches to deprivation cover a wider range of contents.
- Who or what is deprived? Is the focus of attention the individual; the social group (in some sense different from their constituent individuals); other social or quasi-social configurations, such as people of a certain ethnicity, religion or nationality; or, as is the case in some current social policy applications, a geographical area? The decision as to who or what may be deprived will influence the choice of components to be measured.

The extensive academic literature on theories of deprivation (Section 11) may help in making these decisions. There are also several empirical routes for defining deprivation, three of which are summarised below.

The *relative deprivation approach*: is survey based. Respondents are asked to specify which of a list of items they believe are essentials, and then asked whether or not they themselves have access to them. This approach, first used in Britain by Mack and Lansley [191], has been used in a number of industrialised countries and in at least one developing country [192].

The *attitudinal approach*: is also survey based, in which respondents are asked to estimate income levels which they consider 'just enough to make ends meet', 'insufficient', or on which they could only 'manage with some difficulty'.

The *budget standard approach*: uses data about society's current standards and patterns of behaviour and combines them into a detailed costing of the components of a minimally adequate level of living. All the budgets distinguish between what are called 'budget standard costs' which comprise food, clothing, personal care, household goods and services and leisure; and 'variable costs', which include housing, council tax, fuel, transport, NHS charges, insurance, debts/fines/maintenance orders, job-related costs, seeking-work costs, pets, alcohol, tobacco and charitable donations (Box 19).

5.1.4 Types of Data Source to Use in an Index

Until the mid-1990s, the lack of any official data set on income, wealth or means-tested benefits meant that it was impossible to analyse poverty or financial deprivation in the U.K. without either conducting special surveys or using proxies for poverty, such as car ownership, overcrowding and

Box 19

Two main versions of the budget approach

- The first method was used by Seebohm Rowntree and, more recently, by the Family Budget Unit (FBU). *It endeavours to include and cost a family's whole purchase given the prevailing patterns of consumption amongst the poor. The FBU has attempted to cost all the components of a typical family budget in the 1990s, first at a 'modest but adequate' (MBA) level, then at a lower level, 'low cost but acceptable' (LCA). For LCA budgets, the FBU distinguishes between variable costs (like housing, fuel, transport and children) and standard costs over which the families have more control (like food and clothing).*
- The second method is used by the U.S. National Research Council Panel on Poverty and Family Assistance. *It restricts the budget to core items like food, clothing, utilities; the costs of which are rounded up by a multiplier.*

lack of amenities. Most attempts to measure deprivation made extensive use of proxy measures and the main source of data was the Decennial Census.

Many of the better known U.K. indexes of deprivation use Census data. However, non-Census data sources are increasingly available, especially data from the benefits system, such as claimant counts. These have the advantage of being regularly updated, and of measuring income (at least for the poorest groups) more satisfactorily than the Census proxies. A new generation of indexes are being developed that use combinations of Census and administrative data, or in a few cases, entirely administrative data. The pressure to include administrative data that can be regularly updated is particularly strong as indexes are increasingly used for resource allocation. Indexes that use census variables rely on data that can be a decade old.

There is a perennial problem of finding and acquiring data that address certain aspects of deprivation, especially crime, housing and the environment. Often these data are only publicly available at high levels of aggregation. Lower level data may be difficult to access in order to protect individual or commercial confidentiality and may be costly. Much data from national surveys are simply not available for small areas because the values are based on too few cases to be reliable. In fact, many interesting aspects of deprivation cannot be investigated at a sub-local authority level because of the lack of reliable small area data.

One of the main advantages of the Decennial Census is the capacity to deliver small area data. Data from the 1991 Census data for England and

Wales are available to both ward and ED level with two exceptions: certain tables are only included in the Local Base Statistics (LBS) set and not the Small Area Statistics (SAS) set (the LBS tables are only available down to ward level); and very small cell counts are 'Barnardised' in both series – in that −1, 0, or +1 are added randomly to cell counts in order to avoid any possibility of individuals or households being identified.

Results for the 2001 Census have been generated for local authority areas and wards, but a new lower level set of building blocks has been produced. These output areas (OAs) are constructed from contiguous postcodes to create areas with a target of 100–125 households. Their boundaries are drawn in order to maximise the homogeneity of populations within the OAs.

Much of the non-Census data being incorporated in deprivation indexes has not been collected with full postcodes (benefits data are an exception), and is only reported for larger areas than those to which most indexes refer. Some of the indicators in the Index of Multiple Deprivation-2004 (ODPM) suffer from this problem. Although ward level values are published for this index, not all of its components are based on data that are genuinely available at ward level. Various modelling or apportioning procedures have had to be used to estimate ward level values for these components.

5.2 Selecting an Index of Deprivation

There are a number of questions to bear in mind when choosing or developing indexes of deprivation:

- Does the indicator cover a suitable range of topics for its intended purpose?
- Do its component indicators and the associated data sources refer to the correct period in time?
- Are the components suitably transformed and what is the justification for any weights that are used to produce domain or overall scores?
- Have the properties of the instrument been tested statistically and are the results helpful in deciding on the appropriateness of the index for its intended purpose?
- Are there suitable data to compute index values for the intended application? If so, is it important that these are regularly updated?

5.3 The Properties of Deprivation Indexes

Methods for testing and evaluating indicators are discussed in detail in Section 7. Reliability and validity are the two most often used in relation to indexes of deprivation, but neither are particularly easy to apply to these measures. Moreover, it is important to remember that passing various statistical tests is no guarantee of the suitability of an index for a given application.

5.3.1 Reliability

Lee et al. [193] tested the reliability of a batch of Census-based deprivation indexes using the sample of anonymised records which provides a set of individual level data from the 1991 Census. As expected, they found that the instruments with the narrowest range of questions had the most statistical reliability. Four of the indexes had values of Chronbach's alpha of between 0.4 and 0.5 – the index with the widest range of content (the Jarman Index) returned a value of 0.05. The suggested optimum values are between 0.7 and 0.9 (the meaning of these tests are discussed in Section 7) [194]. For additional reading on statistical tests for reliability we recommend Streiner and Norman [195] and Nunnally [196].

Although such tests of reliability are helpful, it is unclear whether they should be used as the major criteria for comparing and choosing measures. Different applications address different notions of deprivation, thus measures may need to have different statistical properties. Questions to ask prior to statistical testing that will influence the interpretation of those tests, include: do we think that deprivation (for the purpose of the intended application) is uni- or multi-dimensional, and how far do we want the measuring instrument to reflect any multi-dimensionality? Having distinct dimensions within an instrument may increase the likelihood that values of the overall score will be sensitive to changes in values of the individual components, which not only increase statistical unreliability (the same measures score differently on two occasions) but may result in an overall volatility, undesirable for applications such as resource allocation.

5.3.2 Validity

Tests of validity try to judge whether an instrument measures what it should be measuring. Such tests therefore require a prior view of what should be measured. Typically, this will require decisions on which aspects of deprivation should be covered, what principle of deprivation is most relevant and whether the measures should apply to all people and places or only certain groups and areas. Having drawn up a specification for the measure, the tests for validity might then involve questions as:

- Does an index concentrate on social as well as, or instead of material dimensions?
- Is an index more appropriate to urban rather than rural areas? (Box 20)
- Is an index biased towards certain age groups? (Box 21)

Box 20

Rural or urban bias in an index?

Most measures of deprivation focus on urban rather than rural phenomena. In the most extreme instances they include circumstances that are irrelevant to rural conditions, such as the proportion of children living in flats. The problems of deprivation in rural areas have been widely discussed and it has been argued that indexes for rural use should include categories such as transport costs and poverty amongst those in low paid employment. Also circumstances such as multiple car ownership have a very different meaning in rural and urban areas. The Oxford Group (Social Disadvantage Research Centre) have tried to include categories that relate to rural deprivation in their Index of Multiple Deprivation-2004 and the Welsh IMD. Items of particular interest are: access to a post office, large food shops, a GP, and a primary school.

Box 21

Youth or older age

Several authors have noted that that some indexes tend to be less valid or reliable as measures of deprivation amongst older people. O'Reilly [197] notes that "the Acheson report acknowledged that there is a lack of routinely collected reliable data on social class or other markers of social economic status in people after the age of retirement". The dependence of most Census-based indexes of deprivation on measures such as class and unemployment partially masks the circumstances of older people. This is especially unhelpful when the indexes are being related to health or healthcare utilisation as to poverty and deprivation amongst older people, who have poorer health and higher healthcare use.

O'Reilly concludes that "many of the commonly used indicators of deprivation are poorly suited to studying inequalities in health in older people," and that the "uptake of income support offers many conceptual and pragmatic advantages over conventional indicators and demonstrates steeper social gradients at older ages than previously thought". Jones and Cameron [198]

So far we have mainly considered qualitative tests for validity. However, there are also statistical approaches, mostly of two types: those that test the index against an accepted measure of the phenomenon (criterion validity) and those that compute correlations between the index and phenomenon the index is intended to measure (construct validity).

Although there is considerable difficulty applying tests for criterion validity, two main U.K. indexes of deprivation, the Breadline and Jarman Indexes have been validated in this way. Lee et al. note that few of the other deprivation indexes used in the U.K. actually claim to have any systematic theoretical basis or to be explicitly validated against a theoretical model of poverty or deprivation [193].

They also explore construct validity by computing correlations between the 10 indexes they review and three factors – estimated mean earnings (based on the Census results for the distribution of occupations and the 1991 New Earnings Survey); under 64 SMRs; and standardised illness ratios (from the Census question on Limiting Long-term Illness (LLTI)). Based on largely statistical assessments, their main conclusions on reliability and validity were two-fold [193]:

- "Socdep, Breadline and Scotdep are, on average the most valid. Scotdep is the most accurate (in respect of the validating criteria), but is also the most unreliable".
- "If the research demands the highest possible levels of accuracy, such as when to measure how many poor wards there are in a region then Scotdep is the best index. However, if a problem requires both a valid and reliable result, such as when trying to rank the poorest wards in a region, then Breadline is clearly the best index. If the research problem is just to look at a specific aspect of deprivation, then in this specialised case Socdep would be the best index to use".

These are helpful judgements, but they need to be treated cautiously. As previously noted, reliability is not an unambiguously good property for an index of deprivation. Moreover, tests for validity, such as those used by Lee et al. only show that 'valid' indexes are highly (linearly) correlated with premature death, self-report illness and an indirect measure of income amongst the employed.

5.3.3 The Index Becomes the Phenomenon

As administrative data sources are becoming more widely available, they are encouraging a trend towards more extensive and complicated measures. As the differences between measures increase, the meaning of what they measure becomes increasingly important. Although they are 'measures of deprivation' is it unclear that they all address the same phenomenon, and it may be the differences are becoming more important than the similarities. Results can differ markedly when different measures are used for the same application – clearly a cause for concern if the application is resource allocation. Increasingly, it is important to understand why an index produces certain results. This is not always easy, given the complexity of some indexes (Sections 10 and 11 address the ways in which choice of indicators and study design can influence the results).

Although a proliferation of indexes may cause confusion, the domination by a single index may be equally undesirable if its definition starts to substitute for the meaning of the concept for which it is only an imperfect estimate. This tendency for a measure to appropriate the meaning of the construct is sometimes known as 'reification'. This tendency is common place, for example it is more common to say 'the ten most deprived local authorities', rather than 'the authorities with the top ten scores on the Index of Multiple Deprivation-2004'. Reification can have undesirable consequences – not least that users may forget to ask what the measurements mean and become less alert to the possibility of alternatives. This lack of conceptual scrutiny may encourage the assumption that the phenomenon being measured has some of the properties of the index. For example, if the devisors have decided to give a particularly heavy weighting to the housing components of the index, it may subsequently be assumed, from the results of using the index, that housing conditions are a key part of deprivation; or if an index includes a measure of the proportion in an ethnic minority population, that ethnicity and deprivation are inextricably linked. Several of these dangers are discussed in Section 7.

5.4 Sources of Further Information – Reviews of Indexes and Their Properties

There are relatively few attempts to compare and contrast the various indexes. One of the more thorough exceptions is the previously mentioned study by Lee Murie and Gordon [199]. It compares 10 indexes, considering their theoretical bases, their components, their methods of combination and the reasons why they may produce different results. It is an excellent source for anyone wanting more detail. Another useful reference prepared for the Policy Action Team (PAT18) is available from the Cabinet Office website and the South West Public Health Observatory site. A third paper by Carstairs and Morris [6] compares the properties of Scotdep with several other Census-based indicators.

The guide to the ONS Classification of Local and Health Authorities of Great Britain is another excellent source of material on methods of area classification. It is available from the National Statistics website.

5.5 Conclusion and Summary of Key Issues Concerning Indexes of Deprivation

Measurements of inequality are often based on indexes of deprivation, but using indexes is not as easy or straightforward as many would like to believe. There are a number of key issues surrounding their use:

- Different indexes of deprivation may not be measuring the same thing.
- Although there are different theoretical definitions of 'deprivation', few of these have been used as the basis for specific indicators.
- Indicators tend to be built from patchy components, because they are limited to what data are actually available.
- There is a risk of 'reification' when an indicator is widely used, especially when it becomes the standard.
- Some existing indicators are biased towards urban conditions, and may discriminate against elderly people.
- Indexes cannot always all be computed for small area bases.
- There is a tendency to reduce reliance on data from Decennial Censuses in favour of data from administrative sources and more frequent surveys, making historical comparison difficult.

SECTION 6

A SELECTION OF INDEXES OF MULTIPLE DEPRIVATION

6.1 Indexes from Census or Administrative Data?

This section introduces most of the better-known indexes of multiple deprivation, divided into those that are exclusively census-based and those that also incorporate other sources. In Section 5, it was noted that the current trend is to move from purely Census-based indicators to those using both of Census and administrative data. Over the past few years there has been considerable lobbying for greater use of non-Census sources, especially from large urban and metropolitan areas. High population mobility and economic pressures can lead to major and rapid social change such that measures of deprivation based on data from the Decennial Censuses fail to identify areas with new problems. This lobbying has been inspired by the increased use of deprivation scores in targeting regeneration and other strategic funds and the release of small area means-tested and other benefits data, including unemployment claimant counts – the closest we have to a national measure of poverty.

In England and Wales, the 'Oxford Group' at The Social Disadvantage Research Centre at the University of Oxford is a major developer of the new generation of indexes. They are responsible for the IMD 2000/2004 and the Welsh IMD and were commissioned, jointly with the South East Public Health Observatory, to produce the Health Poverty Index (HPI).

In Scotland, Kearns et al. [200] have developed an index mainly based on non-Census data. A number of resource allocation formulae for the NHS already use unemployment and income support data.

The release of the 2001 Census results may revive the interest in using Census variables since it provides new and highly flexible low level OAs and powerful mapping capabilities. At the same time, there will be problems for some of the long-established instruments, such as the Jarman Index, as these use variables that did not have precise equivalents in the 2001 Census.

It will be interesting to see whether the enthusiasm for up-to-the-minute data for resource allocation begins to wane when it becomes a major determinant of annual funding. At present, most of the equations using these data direct the allocations of relatively small amounts of health and local authority expenditure. When large proportions of the allocations are determined by current data allocations may vary so greatly from year to year that it becomes difficult to maintain core services. Although the need for some services may be directly related to short-term fluctuations in levels of unemployment or levels of benefit claims, it may not be as relevant for many health and other public services.

Many of the causes of expressed morbidity are not always contemporaneous but are often the consequence of lifetime exposure. The health and disease status of an individual of 60 is the result of a lifelong exposure to environmental, lifestyle and genetic factors. Therefore, data reflecting the conditions of the area 10 years ago may conceivably be a better proxy for health than current data, at least for those who stay in the area. The advantage of recent data is that it is more likely to refer to the current residents rather than that it is more relevant to the measurement of their need for healthcare.

There are other potential problems with the non-Census sources and material employed in the Oxford Indexes. One problem is its relative inaccessibility to local users. Although domain scores are available for the IMD and the Welsh IMD, values for the component variables are not released on a small area basis. Some of these variables are difficult for local authorities to estimate as they are based on elaborate modelling-down procedures using data from national surveys, or complex mapping and apportioning techniques. Some of these data may be too expensive for purchase by local authorities and other local agencies. Also issues of commercial secrecy and ethics relating to fully postcoded data may impede or preclude local access to some of the more useful sources.

6.2 Census-based Indexes

The components of eight indexes based on Census data are briefly described in Table 6.1.

The IMD

The IMD 2000 is an attempt to develop an index from Census variables to predict low income prior to the national availability of income support data. Income support data obtained from Oldham and Oxford, were regressed against a set of Census variables. The resulting equation contains seven Census variables (Table 6.1) to predict areas of low income.

The Jarman Index

This well-known index followed the Acheson committee's call for evidence on the areas in which there was most difficulty providing effective primary care.

Table 6.1. *Components of Census-based indexes*

Variables	*Jarman (UPA8)*	*Townsend*	*Scotdep*	*Socdep*	*Matdep*	*DoE91 ED ward and district*	*Breadline*	*Oxford (IMD)*
Unemployment	X	X	X (male)	X		X	X	X (male)
Youth unemployment				X				
Economically inactive								X
Children in poor households						X		
Children aged under 5	X							
Lone parents	X			X			X	X
Overcrowding	X	X	X		X	X		X
Lacking amenities					X	X		
Lack central heating					X			
Low social class	X		X				X	
Single pensioner	X			X				
No car		X	X		X	X	X	
LA rental								X
All rental (not owner occ)		X					X	
Owner occupiers								X
Children living in flats						X		
Born new commonwealth	X							X
Residential mobility	X							
Self-report long-term limiting illness				X			X	
Single dependent pensioner households				X				

A pilot survey was conducted on 100 London GPs, asking what services and socio-demographic factors put most pressure on their workload. The final questionnaire was distributed to 1 in 10 of all GPs. It asked them to rate the relative importance of 13 social factors (identified in the pilot), including unemployment, poor housing, and single parent households, and eight service factors, such as long out-patient waiting times, high percentage of single-handed GPs and low local authority expenditure on home help.

The index was constructed from the results, with two major omissions. All the service factors were excluded, partly because they were thought to be sensitive to changes in local and national policy and NHS management, and also that there were no relevant data at small area level. Several important social variables were also dropped, including the highest rated factor (the proportion of the population aged over 65) and transport difficulties in visiting patients. These variables were omitted because the existing GP remuneration scheme already took them into account. Crime rate was excluded because there was no suitable Census variable or proxy. Several other variables were excluded because of differences between the 1971 and 1981 Census definitions. The final version of the index is based on eight variables (see Table 6.1).

All eight are derived from 1991 Census, but are subject to algebraic translations to standardise and otherwise improve their distributional properties. The transformed variables are combined using weights derived from the GP ratings in the 1981 National Survey of GPs.

The index is still widely used and was used in the methods for computing GP remuneration until last year. That it is still described as the UPA8 (the 8-item Underprivileged Area Score) is a reminder of the ambiguity that surrounds its development. The question is whether it is a measure of deprivation or of the factors that GPs perceive as impacting on their workload, excluding those that were already incorporated in the remuneration scheme in 1981. Strictly speaking, it is the latter. Although it was not designed as a measure of deprivation, it is of interest in measuring health inequalities because it has been found to be a good predictor of some types of healthcare utilization.

The Townsend Index

The Townsend Index [201] is an unweighted combination of four variables, representing a best attempt to measure material deprivation with the range of data available from the 1981 and 1991 Censuses. The four variables cover: lack of access to good housing (having to rent and live in overcrowded conditions), lack of material possessions, lack of access to private transport (no car) and unemployment.

Until the recent availability of means-tested benefits' data, the Townsend Index was a popular choice for studies wanting to compare levels of morbidity and mortality in different economic groups. Townsend himself uses the index for this purpose in an analysis of health inequalities in the north of England [202].

Scotdep

Scotdep is quite closely related to the Townsend Index in its intentions; it was developed by Carstairs and Morris for the analysis of Scottish health data and health inequalities [203,204]. In a subsequent comparison with four other indexes, its authors conclude that their formula, together with the Townsend Index, are the best of this group at predicting variations in health. As with Townsend, Scotdep is entirely Census-based. The two indexes have three variables in common: unemployment, no car and overcrowding. For the fourth variable, Scotdep replaces rented housing with low social class because the proportion of social rented housing in Scotland was sufficiently high to blunt its sensitivity. Statistically, Scotdep is also similar to Townsend: an unweighted combination of four standardised variables. Its calculation is even simpler as it lacks the log transformation that Townsend uses to reduce the skewness of unemployment and overcrowding.

Matdep and Socdep

Gordon and Forrest's [190] approach to index construction received considerable attention amongst local authorities following the 1993 release of the small area results from the 1991 Census. The two indexes described here reflect the Townsend distinction between material and social deprivation. The components of Matdep will be familiar to those who use either the Townsend Index or Scotdep: overcrowding, lack of amenities (no bath or shower and/or no inside WC and/ no central heating), and no car. The method of calculation is also similar: an unweighted combination of Z scores. The main differences are that a higher proportion of Matdep's components refer to housing conditions and that lack of car ownership is the main proxy for income. As Carstairs and Morris note: "one single indicator (no car) emerges as a variable which performs well in explaining variations in health measures" [205].

The relation between lack of car ownership and poor health is unsurprising given the positive correlation with poverty and age. However, these effects are strongest in urban areas and indexes that exclusively use car ownership as the economic proxy may not always be valid for use in rural areas or for rural urban comparisons.

Socdep is an interesting collection of Census variables that is particularly relevant to predicting the need for local authority services, especially social services. It has six unweighted components, the proportion of: unemployed persons, unemployed youth, lone parents, single pensioners, households with at least one person with LLTI, and households with no member without LLTI.

The Breadline (Britain) Index

This index is made up of Census variables, but was developed by Gordon [199] from an individual and household level analysis of the data from the Breadline Britain survey. The method of derivation makes this index particularly easy to interpret. The aim of the index is to predict which households are 'poor' by using variables from the survey that are also present in the 1991 Census. The analysis of the Breadline Britain survey developed a definition of a poor household – one that is unable to afford three or more of 32 items that are regarded as necessities by 50% or more of respondents.

Variables from the survey are used as the independents in a logistic regression to predict whether or not a household is defined as poor by the above criterion. Because these variables are also present in the 1991 Census, the results of the regression can be used to predict levels of poverty anywhere in Britain. Moreover, the score can be interpreted as a prediction of the proportion of poor households.

The work has received considerable attention and there have been some local replications. Saunders [206] repeated Gordon's approach on a smaller scale with data from the Breadline Greenwich (a south London Borough) survey. Results were similar to Gordon's national analyses except for some differences in the weightings of the variables. Saunders concludes that replicating the Breadline survey locally can be a good basis for developing accurate and meaningful indicators of local deprivation.

6.3 Indexes with a Majority of Non-Census Components

Five indexes are described: Scottish Area Deprivation Index, The Index of Multiple Deprivation-2004, The Welsh IMD, HPI and the Arbuthnot Index.

The Scottish Area Deprivation Index

Developed by Kearns et al. [200] in the mid-1990s , this was a significant attempt to produce an index from non-Census data. Six domains were chosen on theoretical grounds as representing the main dimensions of deprivation (in urban areas). The choice of variables was largely governed by data availability at the post code level. Generally only two or three variables could be found for each domain and these were reduced to a single variable by a combination of correlational criteria and factor analysis. The final variables are shown in Table 6.2. The index is the unweighted sum of signed logged chi-squared transformed variables. Despite being based on non-Census variables, the Scottish Area Deprivation Index closely correlated with Census-based indexes (Table 6.3).

Table 6.2. *Components of Scottish Area Deprivation Index*

Domain	*Indicator*	*Source*
Housing	Overcrowding	Census
Health/morbidity	SMR 0–64 year olds	ONS
Education	Non-participation in higher education	Scottish DoE
Crime	House contents insurance rating	Four insurance companies
Unemployment	Unemployment claimant count	
Poverty	Income support recipients	

Table 6.3. *Correlation of Scottish Area Deprivation Index with several Census-based indexes*

	Jarman	*Matdep*	*IMD*	*Carstairs*	*Townsend*
Matdep	0.66				
Oxford	0.81	0.69			
Carstairs	0.78	0.64	0.84		
Townsend	0.82	0.69	0.90	0.86	
New Scottish	0.77	0.63	0.82	0.78	0.84

Source: from Kearns et al. [200] p. 1549.

The IMD-2000/2004 (ODPM) and Welsh IMD

These indexes represent the most ambitious attempts to date to produce multi-dimensional indexes of deprivation for use at small area level in the U.K. Although they use different sets of variables (and therefore their results are not comparable) there are sufficient similarities in their methods of development and construction to discuss these together.

The indexes were developed for various reasons, inlcuding the need to rank areas in order to target regeneration funds, and modelling levels of deprivation to support both national and local policy. These indexes are intended equally for LAs to use in order to understand and address local patterns of deprivation, as well as for national government to assign resources to LAs (or to other areas with special needs).

The development of both indexes included a series of consultations on the constituent domains and variables.

Ward level values for both the IMD 2000 and 2004 (ODPM) and Welsh indicators and their domains (but not all their constituent variables) are available on the ONS Neighbourhood Statistics website. The method of construction is principally normative. The intention was that the period of consultation should provide more or less consensual judgements on the choice of constituent domains and variables.

The several reports on the indexes provide useful commentary on the technical feasibility of getting suitable ward-level data. A second round of consultation invited comments on the more promising variables and the reasons for excluding several interesting candidates (the full list of indicators in these indexes is shown in Table 6.4). At this stage in the consultation, proposals were floated for weighting the variables. Two levels of weighting are required. First, to combine the constituent variables into domain scores and second to combine the domain scores into an overall index score. The second is the simpler to describe as it involves normatively derived weights and does not attempt to use statistical techniques such as factor analysis or validation against external variables. Two reasons are given for not using equal weights for all domains: first, the consensus of both the literature and of the project commissioners, that income and employment should carry more weight than the others; second, the domains with the more robust scores should be weighted more than the rest.

The Indexes of Deprivation 2004 (ID 2004) are measures of deprivation for every Super Output Area and local authority area in England. They combine a number of indicators across seven domains (Income, Employment, Heath deprivation and Disability, Education, Skills and Training deprivation, Barriers to Housing and Services, Living Environment deprivation and Crime) into a single deprivation score and rank for each area. There are also six summary measures for County Councils, an Income Deprivation Affecting Children Index, and an Income Deprivation Affecting Older People Index.

The development of both indexes is impressive in the range of techniques employed to estimate, improve and combine the values of the component variables. Most of the methods are described in Section 7. The methods included the following:

- *Shrinkage techniques* for improving reliability of area values with small nominators and denominators applied to most of the variables in the index, instead of the more commonly used signed chi-squared approach.
- *Modelling down and apportioning strategies* to estimate small area values for variables that could only be obtained for larger areas.
- *Factor analysis* for combining variables that are not in the form of simple counts. The analysis provides a set of weights to generate factor scores and may suggest that some variables should be dropped.

The Health Poverty Index

The NHS Plan specifically mentions the development of a HPI as one of the tools for addressing inequalities in health and service provision. Eleven consultative workshops were held in 2001 to investigate the types of health poverty measurement that were already taking place, and collect suggestions for the structure and components of a new index.

Following the publication of the Health Poverty Index Scoping Project (July 2001), the Department of Health commissioned the South East Public Health Observatory in collaboration with the Social Disadvantage Research Centre of the Department of Social Policy and Social Work (Oxford University) to develop the HPI. A website for consultation was launched around March 2003 and modified in response to comments received from registered users and an expert user advisory group. It is available as an online tool to make comparisons between areas (by local authority and primary care trusts) or groups (http://www.hpi.org.uk).

The Arbuthnot Index

The Arbuthnot Index may have a major impact on the distribution of healthcare resources in Scotland. It originates in the 'Fair Shares for All' programme or 'The National Review of Resource Allocation' that was established in 1997 to advise on methods of allocating NHS resources between the Scottish Health Boards. The review proposed many separate formulae for predicting the consequences of population characteristics on the need for different types of NHS activities. At the consultation stage, these formulae were thought to be too complicated, so there was pressure to find a single index that might be a simpler predictor of need.

Appendix F to the 'Fair Shares For All' report states that: "four indicators were found to be significantly more successful than other indicators in explaining the differences observed in the use of services between postcode areas". The indicators are:

- The SMR among people aged 0–64 averaged over a 5-year period.
- The proportion of households having two or more deprivation indicators.
- The proportion of the population aged 65 and over claiming income support.

The indicators based on mortality rates, unemployment and income support are available annually, while the indicator of deprived households is taken from the Census. The index is the unweighted sum of the *Z* scores of the four variables. It appears that the intention is to regress the values of this index against healthcare utilisation data for different types of health services and thereby produce a small set of equations (with the same independent variables) that can be used to compute the extent to which resource allocation has to be weighted for population life circumstances and morbidity (Table 6.4).

Table 6.4. Components of the IMD 2000/2004 and Welsh IMD

Components	IMD	Welsh IMD	Level	Source
Employment				
Unemployed claimant count (averaged to overcome seasonal years)	X	X	W	JUVOS, ONS
People out of work, but in TEC delivered government supported training	X		W	DfEE
People aged 18–24 on new deal options	X	X	W	DfEE/ES
Incapacity benefit recipients aged 16–59	X	X	W	DSS
Severe disability allowance recipients aged 16–59	X	X	W	DSS
Health and disability				
Comparative MRs under 65	X	X	H	ONS
Attendance allowance (above 65s) DLA (below 65s)	X	X	W	DSS
People aged 16–59 receiving incapacity benefit or severe disablement allowance	X	X	W	DSS
Limiting long-term illness (self-report) – age–sex standardised	X	X	W	Census
Low birth weight	X	X	W	ONS
Education, skills and training				
Working age adults with no qualifications (only at UA level)	X	X	M	LFS
Persons aged 16–18 not in fulltime education (computed from child benefit data)	X	X	W	DSS
Proportion of people aged 17 and above who have applied (unsuccessfully) for higher education	X	X	W	UCAS
Key stage 2 primary school education data (only available for school catchment areas – reassigned to Edivs using GIS techniques	X	X	M	DfEE
Primary school children with English as a second language	X		M	DfEE
Absenteeism at primary level (all absences)	X		M	DfEE

(Continued)

Table 6.4. *(Continued)*

Components	*IMD*	*Welsh IMD*	*Level*	*Source*
Housing				
Homeless households in temporary accommodation	X		M	LA HIP returns
Overcrowded households	X		W	Census
Poor private sector housing – modelled from 1996 English house condition survey with RESIDATA	X		M	EHCS/ RESIDATA
Proportion of housing in disrepair (1998 Welsh House Condition Survey)		X	M	WHCS
Proportion of houses w/o central heating (1998 Welsh House Condition Survey)		X	M	WHCS
Proportion of housing w/o roof/loft insulation (1998 Welsh House Condition Survey)		X	M	WHCS
Geographical access to services by those on low income				
Access to a post office	X	X	W	GPO(PO Counters)
Access to large food shops	X	X	W	Data consultancy
Access to a GP	X	X	W	NHS, BMA
Access to a primary school	X		W	DfEE
Access to accident and emergency hospital facilities (Welsh ambulance services NHS Trust)		X	W	WAST
Income				
Adults in income support households	X	X	W	DSS
Children in income support households	X	X	W	DSS
Adults in income based job seekers allowance households	X	X	W	DSS
Children in income-based job seekers allowance households	X	X	W	DSS
Adults in family credit households	X	X	W	DSS
Children in family credit households	X	X	W	DSS
Adults in disability working allowance households	X	X	W	DSS
Children in disability working allowance households	X	X	W	DSS

(*Continued*)

Table 6.4. (Continued)

Components	*IMD*	*Welsh IMD*	*Level*	*Source*
Non-earning, non-IS pensioner and disabled council tax benefit recipients (DSS) apportioned to wards	X		M	DSS
People in HB/CTB households who are not in receipt of income support, JSA(IB) or family credit/working families tax credit (HBMS)		X	WM	

Note: W, ward level data (electoral division in Wales); M, higher level data that has been modelled down or apportioned to ward level; H, higher level data applied unmodified to wards; WM, ward level data with modelling used to fill some gaps in supply.

6.4 Geo-classification and Other Area Classification Systems

Though not primarily designed to measure deprivation or poverty, there are several widely used classifications that distinguish areas by their types of housing and/or populations. At least one of the classifications, Super-Profiles, provides a ranking of types roughly corresponding to levels of disposable income.

The Office for National Statistics Area Classification

This classification "provides a simple indicator of the characteristics of areas and the similarity between areas, for comparative or targeting purposes, and a variable for analysis with other data". It is based on 37 socio-economic and demographic variables from the 1991 Census. A stepwise clustering procedure groups similar authorities and results in a three-level classification (for the 406 local authorities) of: 7 families, 15 groups and 27 clusters. Examples of the titles used for the groups include: rural areas, remoter rural, urban fringe, coalfields, ports and industry, and prosperous England.

An attractive feature of this method is that it provides a measure of the distance/difference between authorities and groups of authorities, and that these can be pictorially represented to give an indication of the relationship between the various types.

The classification has recently been re-computed to take account of the changes in local and health authority boundaries. The results are freely available from the ONS website. There is a ward level classification that can be purchased from the same source.

ACORN and SuperProfiles

Two major marketing companies have produced methods for classifying the population of areas to assist in advertising, marketing and product targeting. Both sell products that convert postcodes to their population categories; they also have large databases of the purchasing and life-style patterns of these population groups.

The ACORN system, (www.caci.co.uk) is entirely based on Census data and uses variables such as age, education, SEG, housing tenure and car ownership. The 17 ACORN primary groups are described both in terms of area type (predominately referring to housing stock) and types of resident. For example, Group 4 is “affluent executives, family areas”, and Group 13 is “older people, less prosperous areas”.

The 17 groups are sub-divided into 54 types. For example, Type 5, a subset of Group 1 “wealthy achievers, sub-urban areas”, is described as “mature, well-off suburbs”.

The SuperProfiles system (from CLARITAS) bases its classification on a slightly wider range of sources and uses credit information and market research data in addition to Census variables. It is a three-level system. The most detailed level divides areas into 160 SuperProfile Clusters, which are based on 40 market profile groups, which, themselves are sub-categories of 10 SuperProfile Lifestyles. Examples of these lifestyles are: affluent achievers, thriving greys, hard-pressed families and have-nots.

Both the ACORN and SuperProfile systems have been used to present information on health inequalities. It looks as though the Department of Health has licensed at least one version of the SuperProfile system for internal use. There has been little evaluation of the effectiveness of these profiles as proxies for deprivation. Aveyard et al. [207] considered the relationships between mean birth weight and both Townsend deprivation scores and ranked versions of the SuperProfile Lifestyle and Target Market groups, and found that the SuperProfiles approach may not be suitable for very small-scale work as the analysis was based on sub-ward or enumeration district. Further evaluations would be helpful, as there is considerable interest in using SuperProfiles as a tool for mapping health inequalities.

SECTION 7

INDEXES: PROPERTIES AND PROBLEMS

Following on from Section 5, which introduced using indexes to measure deprivation, and Section 6, which introduced a selection of the better-known indexes, this section examines the construction and properties of indexes, and some of the problems that can arise.

7.1 Introduction

Indexes are one of the basic tools for measuring inequality. They are widely used and new ones continue to be devised. Indexes are available to measure most aspects of health and disease, quality of life and many interpretations of deprivation. They are often employed where there are no simple or direct measures of a phenomenon.

Indexes vary in complexity. They may represent the core phenomenon well, partially or poorly; and a particular index may have properties, including statistical properties, that makes it ideal or quite unsuitable for specific applications.

This section examines the construction and properties of indexes and possible consequences of using them uncritically. The material is relatively technical, but, not excessively statistical. If you require additional statistical details, there are several excellent references which are referred to at various points in the discussion.

The section opens with an example describing the measurement of health with indexes of different levels of complexity. Next there is a more formal summary of the structure and construction of an index, followed by details of the main methods of testing. This section ends with a discussion of the problems that arise if an index is poorly constructed or not suited for its purpose, and what can happen if users forget that an index is only a constructed measure.

7.2 Measuring Disability and Limiting Illness with Indicators and Indexes

This extended example will illustrate the different degrees of complexity of indexes from simple one-component measures, to elaborate multi-level constructions. The example concentrates on how one might measure differences in the incidence of limiting or disabling illness between electoral wards.

Single component indexes

The question on the incidence of disabling illness can be answered with a single item from recent Decennial Censuses. It asks whether each member of the household has a Limiting Long-term Illness (LLTI). This data item is widely used in U.K. health indexes and is often included in both national and local health surveys. When divided by a count of the number of residents in households, it provides an easily computed index of local health, which, in technical terms, is a single component index.[5]

Single domain, multiple component indexes

It can be argued that the Census item on LLTI is too restricted and perhaps too subjective to use on its own. It might be improved if combined with more 'objective' measures, such as the numbers of people claiming state benefits relating to disability (ward level data on disability claimants is available on the ONS neighbourhood statistics website). Such a composite index is more 'objective' than the original single component measurement and also now has a different meaning. However, although it is based on two components or indicators, it still addresses a single domain (incidence of limiting illness).

There are several technical and theoretical issues when constructing domains from more than one component:

- Why choose these two items, rather than other possible measures of (or proxies for) limiting illness? Is there any theoretical or statistical justification for the choice?
- How do we combine the different variables, in this case, data on self-report LLTI and rates of benefit claims?
- Do we transform the variables to have similar values and distributional characteristics?
- Do we weight their relative contribution to an overall score?

---

[5] In practice, one would not usually compare crude rates of LLTI, but would try to adjust for differences in the age–sex composition of the ward populations. Standardising by age and sex is described in Section 3.1.

We can broaden the index further to cover more aspects of (ill)health and its proxies, such as mortality. This combination is similar to the health domain of The Welsh IMD, in which three other items are added to the two we have chosen (Box 22). The five components were selected from a larger group that were suggested by various consultation exercises and literature reviews. The choice was narrowed on practical grounds, such as lack of data at a suitable level, or data that were insufficiently robust (e.g. infant mortality ratio). Other candidate variables, such as the numbers of people using alcohol or drug misuse services, were rejected because their values would be too dependent on the availability of relevant services, and others such as poor dental health amongst children were thought to be too specific to be markers of general health.

Box 22

Components of the health deprivation domain of the Welsh IMD

- Age- and sex-SMRs for people under 65 for 1995–2000.
- People receiving attendance allowance or DSS for 1998.
- People (aged 16–59) receiving incapacity benefit or severe disablement allowance for 1998 and 1999.
- Age- and sex-standardised ratio of LLTI (1991 Census).
- Proportion of births of low birth weight (<2500 g) ONS for 1993–1997.

Clearly, as its authors intend, we now have a measure that tries to measure most aspects of poor general health, albeit limited by data availability.

Even a casual glance at the list of indicators suggests there may be difficulties combining them; not only do they have different metrics – some are rates, others are standardised ratios, but they also contribute unequally to the overall score.

In the case of the Welsh IMD, as there was no a priori (theoretical) basis for combining the items, the devisors used factor analysis to examine the patterns of correlations between the indicators. Unlike the conventional use of factor analysis, where one attempts to identify different factors amongst groups of variables, their interest was in "testing a one-common factor model against the possibility of there being more than one". If other meaningful factors were found, this would suggest that the chosen set of indicators was not measuring a single phenomenon. When the one-factor model was found to be successful, the coefficients of the variables were then used as weights to combine the components into a single domain score.

Multiple domain indexes

So far, we have been regarding health as a single domain (at least for the purpose of measurement) represented by a diverse set of indicators. The multi-dimensional notion of health was discussed in Section 4.3.9 in relation to instruments such as the SF-36 that measure several health domains. In the case of the SF-36 these are: physical functioning; social functioning; energy/vitality; physical impact on social role; emotional impact on social role; mental health; experienced pain; and general health. It is rare to find a health index based on census and administrative data covering the same topics as those based on questionnaires, but such measures could be constructed using, for example, Hospital Episode Statistics (HES).

The domains in multiple deprivation indexes are usually more diverse than different aspects of health. For example, the Welsh IMD has six domains (Box 23), including the health domain discussed above. This is an example of one of the more structurally complex indexes: a multi-domain, multi-component measure.

Box 23

The six domains of the Welsh IMD (and their weightings)

Income deprivation (25%)
Employment deprivation (25%)
Health deprivation and disability (15%)
Education, skills and training deprivation (15%)
Housing deprivation (10%)
Geographical access to services (10%)

By this example, we have tried to illustrate the range of structural complexity found in indexes; these are presented more formally below.

7.3 Key Aspects of the Construction and Structure of Indexes

The basic anatomy of an index

The most elaborate indexes have at least three levels:

- The lowest level made up of the component, sometimes described as an indicator or variable.
- The next level, the domain or dimension, is made up of one or more components.
- The last level is the overall index, comprised of a collection of domains.

Simpler indexes may only have one or two levels. Where there are multiple domains, opinions differ on the value of presenting separate domain scores, or just an overall index score.

Identifying and specifying domains

There are three main methods by which domains are selected:

- From theory. This is relatively rare and relies on the availability of a theory with sufficient detail for them to be translated in to the domains of an index.
- By other normative routes. This ranges from simple consensus to a multi-staged process with various levels of public consultation.
- Through statistical techniques, such as factor analysis. This may involve sifting through large numbers of candidate variables to identify groups that might be interpreted as domains.

Selecting the components of domains

This can be the crucial phase and explains why broadly defined domains are progressively narrowed and redefined by having to work with limited data. The selection of components often involves several stages:

(1) Deciding what would be appropriate items to include in a domain.
(2) Checking data availability.
(3) Checking data reliability and discarding or transforming unreliable sources.
(4) Examining the correlations between components. Statistical techniques such as Cronbach's alpha and factor analysis may also be used to help decide which variables are central to a domain and those that might be excluded or transferred to other domains.

How the components of domains are combined

This will usually involve two stages:

(1) Some type of transformation to give all the components similar distributional characteristics (transforming to a *Z* score is the most common).
(2) Some type of weighting (often using statistical packages).

How the domain scores are combined

Similar methods are used to combine domain scores into an overall index score (Box 24). At this stage it is worth drawing a distinction between indexes, where:

- The weights are derived from statistical techniques.
- The weights are assigned relative importance by index's devisors.

Weights are generally chosen to reflect the relative importance of domains, but other criteria such as data reliability are sometimes used.

Box 24

Welsh IMD: Combination of domain scores into the overall index score

Because the six domain scores are produced different ways and have, different units of measurements, they need to be transformed into a common metric before being combined into an overall value.

The devisors of the scale rejected two of the more conventional methods of transforming to *Z* scores or ranks. Essentially one would rank ward (electoral division) scores, but transform the rank (scores) to an exponential distribution, to re-introduce some measure of the distance between observations that is lost when the scores are converted to ranks.

The relative weights of the domains was decided by various consultative exercises and by reference to literature, rather than by any statistical techniques.

7.4 Testing an Index

7.4.1 Introduction

It is important to establish if an index measures what it is intended to measure. We take it for granted that physical measures such as a ruler or set of scales, will have been tested to certain standards, but most indexes of deprivation have had little systematic testing, in contrast to measures of general health, where there is a small industry devoted to the psychometric testing and validation of measures.

The literature on measures of health demonstrates the importance placed on psychometric approaches to testing. In the case of health questionnaires, this is understandable, given their increasing use in clinical trials and other settings to test the effectiveness of interventions. Nevertheless, there is some concern that the balance has shifted too far towards statistical rather than substantive criteria – that too much attention is paid to tests such as Cronbach's alpha, rather than the meaning of a measure and its relevance to intended applications.

Indexes are usually assessed on three criteria: validity, reliability and responsiveness. Unfortunately, there are many different interpretations of these criteria. For example, Hays and Hadorn [208] argue that responsiveness is better regarded as a form of validity. However, there is agreement on most of the basic principles and those with an interest in the statistical detail should refer to Streiner and Norman [195]; McDowell and Newell [142].

7.4.2 Validity

There are many forms of validity testing; three approaches – content, criterion and construct validity, are most relevant here.

Content validity, as its name suggests, is concerned with the selection of components and domains in an index (or the questions in a health status questionnaire). With a multi-dimensional instrument there are three main requirements:

- The main topic headings (the domains) should be appropriate to the overall aims of the measurement.
- The components of each domain should relate to the definition and aim of that domain.
- The components should be a representative sample of those that might have been chosen, and should give uniform coverage of the full range of each domain.

For questionnaires, the wording should be intelligible to respondents, and unlikely to be misunderstood or offensive.

The simplest methods for content validity is review by expert panels or a pilot with samples of representative respondents. Such assessments are rarely repeated when a questionnaire is in regular use, thus, its users may fail to notice if the instrument needs to be adapted to reflect changes in the phenomenon being measured, and, in the case of questionnaires, cultural changes overtime.

One of the more important reasons for testing for content validity is to assess and improve the reliability of the instrument. Measurements will tend to be more reliable if all the components of an index address the same core concept.

Many appropriate statistical techniques are available for content validity. Multi-trait scaling and factor analysis were employed in developing the SF-36 questionnaire both to eliminate items that were least related to the intended constructs and to test whether response patterns reflected the intended conceptual structure.

The principle of *criterion validity* is derived from the testing of physical instrumentation. The aim is to compare a new instrument against a gold standard for which it will then be a substitute. With physical instrumentation, the measurements from two instruments must be very highly correlated if one is to substitute for another – even values of 0.99 may not be acceptable.

The key principles underlying criterion validity in physical measurement – substitution and interchangeability – are hard to apply to indexes and questionnaires, not least because there are no gold standards and no two instruments seem to be designed to measure the same thing. Nevertheless, there is a great deal of this type of testing in relation to measures of health. It is possible to correlate one measure (such as the SF-36) against another (such as the NHP), or to correlate domains of the measure with single items within the measure itself as shown by Jenkinson et al. [209]. Understandably, the values of the correlations in these comparisons are much lower than those required for one instrument to substitute for another. Consequently, the hypothesis, "is there any evidence that the two instruments are not providing equivalent measurements?" is replaced by the much weaker, "is there any evidence that the measurements are not unrelated?".

A common problem in criterion validity is when there is no gold standard to use as a benchmark. One well-known exception is where several indexes have been validated against a definition of poverty derived from the Breadline Britain Survey. However, it is far more common for validity to be tested by analysing the correlations between the index score and phenomena which are thought to be related to deprivation. For example, Lee et al. [193] compute correlations between the 10 indexes they review and three factors that are either regarded as part or consequences of deprivation (see Section 5.4 for more details).

Construct validity tests for predicted associations. For example, if there are theoretical grounds for believing that perceived general health should be associated with the number of visits to a GP, or levels of self-medication, then this can be formally tested, and, if confirmed, will add to the evidence of construct validity. Trying to confirm plausible associations and disprove the implausible can be a long process. Often, there will be no definitive answers and, at present, there are no formal ways to weigh the overall evidence. Hence, it is unsurprising that tests of construct validity have been criticised for their failure to set formal hypotheses or specify in advance what will represent significant evidence [142]. The whole process is better described as an art than a science.

Reaching conclusions on construct validity is further complicated by the problem that evidence tends to be interpreted in two different ways: to use these associations to test whether the instrument is a good measure of the intended constructs; or to look for associations that will confirm and clarify the constructs themselves. There are major differences of statistical principle here, some of which are discussed by Streiner and Norman [195]. It is also very important to be clear about the different questions being answered by different indexes, and therefore what any given test for construct validity is trying to achieve (Table 7.1).

7.4.3 Reliability

Reliability may be defined as the capacity to produce the same result in precisely the same circumstances. This is a most relevant to physical instrumentation that are used repeatedly, such as thermometers or speedometers. With physical instrumentation, the classic test for reliability is to take repeated measurements in the same conditions. With health status questionnaires, reliability is evaluated by administering the instrument on

Table 7.1. *Indexes and the corresponding questions*

Indexes	*Questions*
Indexes based on death	Who dies?
Excess over 'average'	Excess over 'average'
Relative likelihoods	Relative likelihoods
Mortality rates	
Standardised mortality rates	
Ratio of mortality rates or of Standardised mortality ratios	
Percentage of survivors	Who lives?
Standardised survivorship ratios	
Ratio of survivor rates or of SSRs	
Indexes based on morbidity	
Nottingham health profile	Subjective assessment illness
Symptoms reports	occurrences 'objective' morbidity
Condition and/or disease incidence/prevalence	

two separate occasions, separated by a time interval, anywhere from several days to several months, sufficiently long to minimise memory effects but sufficiently short to reduce the likelihood of health having changed. During this period, there will need to be an independent assessment of changes in health, so respondents whose health has changed can be excluded from the re-test. It is difficult to find suitable controls since most health profiles are unique in what they measure. Measurements used as controls have included single item self-reports of health.

Because, it is hard to apply such procedures to indexes, a variety of indirect tests are used instead. Most of these are based on the assumption that a measure will be reliable if its components are highly inter-correlated. One method, the split-test approach, divides the components of an index or questionnaire in half. A single sample of test data is required, and the correlations between the two halves are computed. This technique is limited to measures that can be split into equivalent halves. This examines the correlations between all the components which are summarised by test statistics such as the KR-20 (Kuder and Richarson formula, 20) and Cronbach's alpha.

Very high reliability is not necessarily good as it may point to redundancy, e.g. several components providing very similar measurements. In such cases, it may be possible to reduce the number of components, making the instrument easier to use. Moreover, high reliability is most likely to be a feature of uni-dimensional measures, so if the instrument is intended to measure a multi-dimensional phenomenon, high reliability may be a sign of a partial measurement.

As with most of these psychometric assessments, the acceptable level of reliability will depend on the application. The most demanding applications are those measuring changes in individual's health or average health scores for small groups.

For more on statistical tests for reliability we recommend Streiner and Norman [195] and Nunnally [196].

7.4.4 *Responsiveness*

Responsiveness denotes the capacity of the instrument to measure difference or change. For example, if the aim is to map demographic variations in health then the ability to detect cross-sectional differences between the health status of different age, gender and condition groups may be sufficient evidence of responsiveness. (See Box 25).

Greater responsiveness is needed for clinical applications where an instrument is required to detect changes in health due to an intervention. Although it may be sufficient to show that the instrument can differentiate between those with different levels of clinical severity for the same condition, more often it will be necessary to demonstrate the ability to detect change due to treatment. In all such tests there is a problem of what should count as significant change. Statistically, significant differences in health status scores may not correspond to clinicians', patients' or carers' views of significant change. Conversely, the changes that these groups regard as significant may not be detected by the instrument.

Responsiveness is normally tested by piloting the instrument in conditions similar to the intended application. However, inspecting the contents of a measure and its distributional properties in the general population may be a guide to its responsiveness. There are two key points to check:

- Are the end-points suitably defined, e.g. will there be 'floor' or 'ceiling' effects?
- Is there good coverage of all the intermediate points – the number and spacing of items and response levels?

Box 25

Responsiveness – a sensitive indicator

An indicator should be sensitive. If someone's socio-economic classification according to an index changes, it is obviously important that this change can be related to a change in that person's position in the social hierarchy, to which the classification refers. Goldthorpe [210] correctly deploys this argument against the use of women's own occupation as the basis for their social class because married women might change their job for life-cycle reasons unrelated to any change in their social position. It is unrealistic to be rigorous here, but it is reasonable to demand that the index be relatively sensitive to 'real' change and relatively stable when there is no 'real' change.

7.5 The Purpose of Testing

One problem with tests such as Cronbach's alpha is the focus on the internal characteristics of an instrument rather than its relationship to the outside world. The statistical testing of indicators should not distract us from asking basic questions about the meaning and performance of indicators or their suitability for specific applications.

For example, depending on the intended use an index of health might:

- Reflect the socio-economic dimension to inequalities in health.
- Reflect the experience of the entire population.
- Be sensitive to changes in the distribution of the population across socio-economic categories.

7.6 Matching the Index to the Application – Example of an Index for Policy Use

Depending on the application, each index requires different properties. For example, what is required of an instrument for policy applications?

An instrument intended for purely academic use may be complex and opaque, however, one intended for policy purposes, such as targeting interventions, should be explicable and defendable to a wider constituency. It should also have:

- *Technical robustness.* It should be based on established analytical techniques and evidence.
- *Transparency.* In general, the index should be simple to understand.
- *Objectivity.* The index should be objective and capable of application to all areas.
- *Plausibility.* It should be capable of reasoned and unambiguous explanation.
- *Freedom from perverse incentives.* It should not create financial incentives that appear to conflict with sensible interventions.
- *Reliability of calculation.* Indexes should use data whose quality is sound, consistent between areas; and available for all areas.
- *Comprehensibility to non-specialists.* The index, should be capable of commonsense justification to non-specialists.
- *Durability.* It should not become quickly outdated.
- *Practicality.* It should be derived — updated in a manageable manner, within the time constraints of the annual financial cycle.

The following characteristics are also highly desirable:

- *Clarity of contribution of constituent indicators and domains.* It is desirable that the relative significance of individual indicators can be quantified.

- *Flexibility.* It should be possible for the index to take account of future changes of responsibilities or structure (e.g. reorganisation or boundary changes).
- *Stability.* Fluctuations in the index arising from fluctuations in data for component indicators should be well founded, rather than a side-effect of limitations in the quality of those data.

It is customary for indexes in policy applications to be frequently reviewed for their capacity to generate policy-relevant results. The criterion of *materiality* comes into play when one is considering changes to existing indexes.

> *Materiality refers to the question of when is it worth introducing an index, or changing an existing index.* The extra technical complexity of the proposed change to the index must be set against the impact of the change on the populations, or resources affected by the indexes.

7.7 Pitfalls and Problems of Using Indexes

7.7.1 Difficulties in Using an Indicator may be a Pointer to Design Problems

If there are difficulties using an instrument it may be that the instrument does not meaningfully reflect the reality it is intended to represent. This can happen in the case of health status questionnaires whose questions seem irrelevant to respondents. It can also happen when classifications over-simplify or misrepresent a phenomenon. In both cases, the questionnaire or index would be invalid for the intended purpose. The rules provided by the OPCS assigning social class to women demonstrate some of these problems (Box 26).

Box 26

Example – how to assign social class to women

The set of rules used by the OPCS for assigning a woman to a category in the Registrar General's Social Class Scale (SCS) varies according to her formal marital status. Thus:

- When married and living with a spouse the woman is classified on the basis of her husband.
- When not living with a spouse and in employment the woman is classified on the basis of her own occupation.
- When not living with a spouse and unemployed, a variety of solutions are adopted.

The convolutions become impenetrable when attempting to classify the single, never-employed woman, who lives on her own and who does not remember her father's occupation.

The problem is that the SCS has violated two technical requirements for a classification: that it should have a *uniform basis*, and that there should be a unique assignment for each case.

In order to provide a unique assignment for each case, the SCS abandons any pretence of having a uniform basis for classification. A woman may be classified either by her own occupation or by that of any near male relative. This is absurd as well as sexist. The SCS may provide an exhaustive as well as a unique classification, but this is only achieved at the expense of the sole purpose for classification.

7.7.2 The Indicator Becomes the Reality

A common problem is to confuse the index with the phenomenon it purports to measure and, as a result, forget that it is only a proxy or partial measure. If the index is widely accepted to the point where there is little questioning of the content and construction, a number of problems can arise, in particular: reification, circularity and impurity. Most of the examples relate to the Registrar General's SCS but the principles apply widely.

Reification

Reification is a common problem. Although a proliferation of indexes may cause confusion, the domination by a single index may be equally undesirable as its operational definition may start to substitute for the meaning of the concept of which it measures. It is especially prevalent in the measurement of self-reported health status, where questions derived from the SF-36 and its shorter versions are now virtually accepted as the lay conception of health.

The same tendency is experienced with measures of deprivation where it is more common to use phrases such as "the ten most deprived local authorities", rather than "the authorities with the top ten scores on the IMD". Reification is likely to lead to forgetfulness – that what is being measured is not deprivation, but a very elaborate combination of factors chosen by a combination of political, theoretical and pragmatic criteria.

Circularity

Forgetting about the properties of the measure and its origins, can lead to circular forms of thinking (Box 27).

Purity

The basis of the classification of the indicator should be 'pure'. For example, the use of tenure *as an index of* 'social class' could not be validated by showing that tenure discriminates access to amenities. A household's tenure directly affects its access to amenities, so we cannot tell if there is any effect upon access to amenities due to 'social class' rather than to

Box 27

The circularity of social class

The indicator proposed should not be *circular*: that is, the evidence produced to justify a causal link should not itself rely on the *explicandum*. For example, a group of people are poor because they are in social class V; they are in social class V because they are poor. Again, the tabulation of educational attainment by social class of head of household shows a typical gradient, but the juxtaposition of observations that: "you are in social class V occupation because you are poorly educated" and "your lack of education is typical of those in social class V," does not constitute the basis of an explanation. This is not trivial. Stevenson [24] (the originator of the social class scheme) fell into this trap when attempting to validate his proposed scheme. The evidence he gives for the validity of SCS as a reflection of social distinctions is that it discriminates mortality. He then claims that, because SCS is a valid mirror of society, we can go on to examine the social process bringing about differential mortality.

tenure. Stevenson [24] was greatly concerned with this problem and accordingly rejected several other possible alternatives to occupation as the basis for his social class classification. He recognised that it was also a problem when using his own occupation-based classification to discriminate mortality, because some jobs were in themselves dangerous, so that the observed differential mortality on the basis of his occupationally based scheme was a combination of a 'social class' effect and occupational risk. This led to his attempt to isolate the 'pure' social class effect by looking at the mortality of wives by the occupational group of their husbands. Whilst the problem of circularity is usually relatively easy to avoid and detect, the problem of 'impurity', like that of 'reification', is much more difficult. On the one hand, detailed and complex measures may extend and confuse the meaning of the core phenomenon, while on the other, over-simple measures, may reduce the intended phenomenon to something trivial and ultimately meaningless.

Testing for purity involves ensuring that indexes have a clear relation to the phenomenon being indicated. Townsend made a similar point,

> "It is, we believe, mistaken to treat being a member of an ethnic minority as part of the definition of deprivation. Even if many among this minority are deprived, some are not and the point is to find out how many are deprived rather than operate as if all were in that condition. It is the form their deprivation takes and not their status which has to be measured" [211].

The measure becomes the explanation

One consequence of reification, especially when linked to circularity, is a confusion between the index and an explanation of the phenomenon being explored.

For example, in many reports, SCS is used not only as an *index* to portray differences but that portrayal is also assumed to constitute an *explanation* of those differences [212]. There are, of course, many reports that do not make that assumption. The Black Report on Inequalities in health [213] is exemplary in this respect, offering four possible explanations for an observed SCS distribution. But, they have difficulty in maintaining the distinction between those four explanations and 'social classes' and the political consequence was that the then hostile government found it easy to ignore their findings (these difficulties were cited by Patrick Jenkin, Secretary of State for Social Services, 1980, as one of the reasons for not endorsing their recommendations), which is a high price to pay for methodological sophistication.

7.7.3 What does a 'quality of life' index mean?

Reification may occur because many multiple domain indicators are so complex that it is near impossible to tell what they are actually measuring, and it is tediously repetitive to list all the components every time an index is referred to. The most complex indicators often purport to measure deceptively simple, 'common-sense' notions, such as deprivation, class, health and, not least, quality of life. If these indexes are used for resource allocation reification can be dangerous. For example, we need to know precisely what interpretation of quality of life has been used in a cost-effectiveness assessment if that assessment concludes that an intervention is not recommended to someone over a certain age. Equally, we need to know what measure of deprivation directs money to one area than another.

The meaning of quality of life measures

The meaning of indexes that claim to represent our own experiences should be subject to special scrutiny, especially if they have policy implications. This may require an investigation of the process of construction of the index, asking how and why critical decisions were made.

Unpacking the meaning of an index is rarely easy – consider the case of a 'quality of life' index (see Section 4.3.10). There are many difficulties with devising an overall quality of life index. In fact, there are two distinct sets of problems: establishing a coherent set of component indicators; and interpreting combinations.

Choice of components

There is no consensus over the components or the weighting procedures to be employed in 'composite' quality of life indexes.

> Whilst everyone wants a certain minimum of conditions, few can agree on the optimum level or combination required.
> Whilst nodding in the direction of consumer sovereignty for choosing and combining components, few have actually attempted to take that position seriously.

There is the counter argument that each of the components is the product of a gradual process out of which some degree of consensus has emerged. But, that argument also is the foundation for the objection that it is an historical consensus. Whether or not such components or weighting are relevant to different populations is important. There is no consensus as to how relevance ought to be measured, nor differences reconciled. If public perceptions are to be an eventual component of their experienced quality of life, then the relative importance of different aspects of their situation must also be essential.

Problems of interpretation – trade-offs are obscured

There is a very close correlation between life expectancy and per capita income at a macro (national) level. The relationship between income and health is not so simple, e.g. isolation of elderly and certain forms of child abuse prevail more in high income nations.

Etzioni and Lehman [212], argued against 'formalistic-aggregative measurement of collective attributes', as with the U.S. Crime Index, which aggregates a broad range of crimes, thus giving the same weight to a murder and a $50 theft.

For many applications it may be important to ensure that although the use of indexes has advantages, we should not lose interest in individuals, and a concern with extremes as well as averages; and should not lump everything together which will tend to produce bland results.

The point is that not only is well-being multi-dimensional, its aspects are incommensurable in that although they are inter-related, they are not substitutable for each other. For example, a sufficient income to ensure good nutrition increases life expectancy, but you cannot compensate early deaths with high income. Although an index, through continued use can be presented as being simple, such as GNP, the underlying presumptions are often quite complex and obscured.

Lack of disaggregation

Few quality of life indexes address distributional aspects of the different components of the 'quality of life' or 'well-being' of particular population groups.

This is principally because of the difficulty of collecting sufficient nationally comparable data to yield meaningful estimates at the community level or for small groups; such indexes can usually only be calculated for highly aggregated and often inappropriate geographic units of analysis.[6]

7.8 Conclusions

Although this section has concentrated on what may seem to be relatively obscure and technical aspects of indexes, the questions covered are increasingly important when indexes are being used to inform decisions on resource allocation, targeting and rationing at every level of government.

Although it is unlikely that there will ever be a perfect index for every (or any) application, it is at least worth trying to ensure that the chosen instrument:

- Is not circular or prone to misinterpretation or reification.
- Provides a uniform basis for a unique assignment for each case.
- Can be derived from easily collectable data in a form which corresponds to the underlying phenomenon.
- Is relatively sensitive to changes or stability in the underlying phenomenon.

It is also worth remembering that there is no such thing as a universally valid or reliable index; that different applications will require different properties, which may be substantive – such as using a transparent index in resource allocation; or technical – such as using an index with sufficient responsiveness to detect the suspected inequality.

Finally, each index comes complete with assumptions and premises, resulting from its methods of construction, the choice of components and any attendant theory. These may not always be obvious, but they will influence the instrument's performance and results. Hence, after any statistical testing, one should always ask "what does an index really mean?"

---

[6] This is also because of confidentiality, where data at small area levels or for small groups are 'Barnardised', that is, -1, 0, or $+1$ are randomly added to the counts.

SECTION 8

DATA SOURCES: AVAILABILITY AND PROBLEMS

Throughout this handbook we have tried to include detailed information on the sources for specific variables within a substantive discussion of those variables. The aim of this section is to provide an overview of some of the major sources of national data that are available for local areas and note some of the potential problems in using these sources. In choosing to concentrate on national data sets, we know that we fail to cover the many valuable sources of local data that will have been compiled by agencies such as Public Health Observatories and local authorities. Although beyond the scope of this handbook, sources of local data may be the best starting point for anyone wanting to make comparisons within relatively limited areas. The difficulty in trying to use such material for more extensive work is the lack of standardisation, especially with respect to methods of data capture, data definitions and data formats.

8.1 Introduction

A surprising range of data relevant to the mapping and analysis of inequalities are becoming increasingly available either free of charge, or for relatively modest payments.

The main suppliers of public data all have searchable websites intended for people who are not already familiar with the range of possible sources.

The range of potentially useful material rapidly reduces if one wants to investigate inequalities at the sub-local authority or sub-health authority level. For example, at electoral ward level, there is no detailed national information on crime or the environment. Many of the more interesting data sources are intended to provide between authority comparisons and are not collected for lower level analyses.

For these reasons, the Decennial Census is still an unparalleled resource.

In addition to the Census, most data used to map inequalities will come from one of three types of sources:

- Postcoded activity data from public services, other government bodies and some commercial organisations.
- Activity data from government and public agencies submitted in aggregate form for periodic returns and performance indicators.
- Data from large-scale surveys.

For the user, the main difference between these is their potential to provide data on small areas. Activity data containing full postcodes are rarely released in order to protect the confidentiality of individuals, but the data may be available aggregated to larger area bases. For example, means-tested benefits data are routinely available at electoral ward and local authority bases, and can be purchased for other areas such as health authorities. A local basket of health indicators has a range of indicators that can be created at a small area level (Section 8.4.11).

8.2 The Area Base

8.2.1 The Desired Base is not Always Available

Aggregated activity data poses a number of problems for small area analyses because it is often only released at the administrative area base of the agency providing the returns. Typical area bases are local authority areas, school catchment populations and police districts. There are several methods for constructing smaller area estimates from these sources. Where the geographical base is uncertain, as in the case of school catchment areas, it may be possible to use mapping techniques to construct hypothetical boundaries between school areas. The devisers of the Index of Multiple Deprivation used these methods to provide ward level estimates of primary school data. Where the geographical base is known, as for many local authority returns, it may be possible to 'model down' this material to, say, ward level. Various statistical techniques can be employed, but they all rely on establishing a relation between the variable that is only available at the higher level and other variables that are also available at the lower level. Typically, if one can show a relationship at local authority level between Census data and the variable of interest, that relationship could be used to apportion the local authority values to sub-authority areas such as electoral wards. The process is fraught with a number of dangers, notably that the relationship used for the apportioning is distorted by the ecological fallacy or authority level supply factors.

There are a number of national household surveys with samples of 20–30,000, which are too small to provide reliable estimates below local authority level. Again, modelling techniques can be used to make ward level estimates. In this section, the modelling will be carried out with the individual level data from the survey, to produce a predictive model that can be used in conjunction with ward level data to provide ward level predictions for the variable of interest. Whenever possible, these models should also be used to model down local authority data, as they avoid many of the problems of models based on higher level data.

Changes in the boundaries of administrative areas can pose difficulties for data users. In the past decade, there have been major changes to local authority, ward, and health area boundaries. These not only pose difficulties for over-time comparisons but also can complicate the linking of contemporary sources. For example, unemployment and benefits claimants counts are currently not released on the same ward bases – the former is based on 1998/1999 ward boundaries and the latter on 1991 ward boundaries (Table 8.1).

Most developers of indexes of deprivation and other potential indicators of inequality are now interested in providing results for areas smaller than local authorities. The advantage of Census data is that they are generally suitable for this purpose. The 1991 Census data for England and Wales are available to both ward and ED level with two exceptions: certain tables are only included in the LBS set and not the SAS set (the LBS tables are only available down to ward level); and very small cell counts are 'Barnardised' – a form of noise is introduced (by adding −1, 0, +1 randomly) to improve anonymity.

Although results for the 2001 Census have been generated for local authority areas and wards, there is a new lower level set of building blocks 'Output Areas', constructed from contiguous postcodes to create areas with

Table 8.1. *Approximate numbers of units and populations in different area bases*

	N in England	*Approximate average population (persons)*
Region	8	6.3M
LAs with respect to social services counties/UAs	149	340K
LAs (districts)	354	150K
Strategic Health Authorities	28	1.8M
Primary Care Organisations	402	120K
Wards	~8640	5.8K
Postcode districts	2260	22K
Postcode sectors	8760	5.7K
Enumeration Districts (Census pre-2001)	110,000 (England and Wales)	490
2001 Census Output Areas	~150,000	100–125 households

a target of 100 to 125 households. Boundaries are drawn in order to maximise the homogeneity of populations within OAs. These new OAs offer the possibility of building customised OAs and there is much interest in using them to construct neighbourhood profiles and provide data to other sub-ward boundaries.

8.2.2 Postcode to Area Translation

At present, the full postcode is the most commonly used standard geographical identifier in administrative data sets, though the Ordnance Survey Grid Reference is becoming a contender. In order to aggregate data to larger areas, some version of the National Postcode Directory (NPD) is required. The NPD is released by ONS (under license from the post office) in a number of formats including different sets of electoral and administrative area codes – a subset of this directory is available throughout the NHS as the NHS postcode directory. Other versions of the postcode directory can be purchased for commercial use. Thousands, or even millions of postcoded records can be converted to some other area code such as ward or local authority in a matter of minutes using these directories, a computer and a statistical package, such as SAS or SPSS. The only drawback, apart from the cost, is that the target data has to be fully postcoded. This is not always the case.

In administrative data sets, postcodes are often missing, incomplete, or invalid, though the quality of postcoding is improving as more systems use automated gazetteers for entering and validating addresses.

In some rural areas, a postcode may contain very few households and only one other piece of information, such as age or ethnicity may uniquely identify individuals. For reasons of confidentiality, there may be objections to releasing fully postcoded data, even if the aim is to aggregate the material.

Another problem can arise when the post office updates and expands the postcode base and administrative databases retain old postcodes that eventually drop-out of the postcode directory. A related problem is that there may be insufficient demand to justify the cost of mapping new postcodes to older area bases, as currently happens with 1991 wards.

Much of the new (non-Census) data being incorporated in deprivation indexes is not available with full postcodes, and is only reported for larger areas than those to which most indexes refer. The Index of Multiple Deprivation-2004 is a case in point. Although ward level values are published for this index, not all of its components are based on data that are genuinely available at ward level or lower. Various modelling or apportioning procedures have had to be used to estimate ward level values for these components.

Currently, there is considerable interest in supplementing or replacing postcodes with grid references as the basic locational identifier in administrative data sets. The Gridlink project is developing a database of grid reference to administrative areas. More details of the project and associated products, such as Ordnance Survey's address-point can be found on the Ordnance Survey website.

8.3 Major National Archives and Sources

Statbase (Office for National Statistics)

The largest collection of freely available data sets is held by the ONS managed Statbase. It has to be noted that many of these sets are small single tables, showing data at regional or local authority level. In fact, many seem to be reformatted tables from official publications.

Neighbourhood Statistics (Office for National Statistics)

This part of the National Statistics website contains ward and LA level data and is likely to be important for anyone wanting to conduct sub-authority analyses of inequality.

Data are free and can be downloaded as Excel sheets or CSV files.

Some key holdings are:

- Ward level data on all domains (though not the separate variables) of the IMD 2004.
- Ward level counts for a large number of means-tested benefits, including income support and family credit and benefits relating to disability.
- Ward level population estimates for 1998 (from the IMD team).

NOMIS

NOMIS is an independently managed database of large-scale data sets, mostly on labour markets, many of which derive from the ONS. It also provides all the LBS tables for the 1991 Census.

Access charges have recently been removed for non-commercial users and most of the NOMIS data sets can now be accessed without charge after a simple registration procedure from ONS.

Some of the key data sets held at NOMIS are:

- All 1991 LBS Census tables at ward and higher levels.
- Current unemployment claimant counts.
- Data from the Labour Force Survey.

The Data Archive

This is by far the largest collection of large (mainly survey-based) data sets in the U.K. As almost all data sets hold individual level data, users have to apply to obtain each data set, giving an account of its intended use, and pay a fee that reflects the handling charge for the type of media required. Note that some of these data sets are too large to fit on single CDs.

One of the strengths of the holding is that most projects funded by Economic and Social Research Council (ESRC) and related government monies have been required to lodge their data and an intelligible coding frame at the archive. It holds material such as the General Households Surveys and large health and lifestyle surveys.

Archive staff will also attempt to trace data sets that are not part of their current holding.

Public Health Observatories

Public Health Observatories were established in each of the nine English regions in order to strengthen the availability and use of information about health at a regional and local level by:

- Monitoring health and disease trends and highlighting areas for action.
- Identifying gaps in health information.
- Advising on methods for health and health inequality impact assessments.
- Drawing together information from different sources in new ways to improve health.
- Evaluating progress by local agencies in improving health and cutting inequality.
- Looking ahead to give early warning of future public health problems.

PHOs increasingly can assist by developing and coordinating analytical expertise across regional and sub-regional networks, sharing methodologies and avoiding duplication of effort as far as possible. PHOs also have a 'critical mass' of analytical skills.

Most of the material produced by the observatories is freely available via their websites. Some of these sites concentrate on reports of the patterning of local health, others also provide data that can be downloaded and re-analysed.

Local basket of health inequalitites indicators

The London Health Observatory has led a project to develop a series of indicators for local use of measuring progress in dealing with inequalities. The local basket of health inequalities indicators was released in October 2003. The basket contains an initial set of 70 indicators. It contains measures of health status or health outcomes, measure of the determinants of health, measures of access to services and process measures. The main purpose of the local basket of indicators is to help support local action to achieve the Government's national inequalities targets for life expectancy and infant mortality. The report on the indicator list and the indicators themselves are available on the London Health Observatory website (www.lho.org.uk).

Other General Sources

Local authorities will employ teams that compile statistics on their area predominately for the purposes of targeting services and other aspects of resource management and allocation. But, as they do not normally regard the public provision of detailed information on sub-authority areas as part of their core function, the range of material that can be found on public websites is both patchy and limited. Nevertheless, they may be prepared to supply detailed information for specific purposes.

Many commercial organisations such as building societies and insurance companies hold important postcode level databases. There are cases of researchers being granted access to these data, but we imagine that uses would be very strictly controlled and likely to be expensive.

8.4 Data Sources on Specific Topics

More details of these sources will be found elsewhere in the handbook, where the topics themselves are discussed. Again, data sets are only mentioned if they have national coverage.

8.4.1 Population Estimates

Population counts are the denominators for many indicators of health and deprivation. During the past decade, ONS has produced rolling population estimates every two years based on the previous Decennial Census (and given some of the doubts of the coverage of the 1991 Census, the estimates were also rooted in the 1981 Census figures). Birth and mortality rates are two of the main factors used to generate the estimates, but they also take account of geographical mobility.

For a number of purposes such as resource allocation, population counts are required in advance of the biennial estimates; to meet this need, ONS provides population projections. In effect, the models used to generate the estimates are run forward, using the last biennial estimate as the base. By this method, projections are prepared for up to three or for years from the last estimate.

The main sources of population estimates and projections are as follows:
On the NOMIS site:

- 1991 Census counts (LBS tables only).
- Resident population estimates for local authorities.
- Ward population estimates are not routinely released by ONS, but the NOMIS site contains the denominators for the Index of Multiple Deprivation-2004.

Other sites/sources

Full versions of the Census data are held at a number of sites and can be also purchased for local use. The English academic community has traditionally accessed Census data via MIDAS – a data set system hosted by the University of Manchester computing service.

The Oxford Group is currently running a national project to improve small area estimates for the numbers of elderly people, a group whose numbers are not always accurately estimated in simple inter-censile projections.

The Compendium of Health Indicators produced by NCHOD for Department of Health includes ONS estimates for health authorities in five year age–sex bands (also on Statbase). It also contains figures for the populations of primary care trusts and groups, based on primary care registrations data, reconciled to ONS estimates and projections at the health authority level.[7]

Results from the 2001 Census were released in late 2002. Access to Census material has radically changed with the 2001 project. Although much of the 1991 material could be got from public websites towards the end of the 1990s, the 2001 results are freely available from the start, though there are handling charges for very large data requests on CD, and additional charges for material specially aggregated to client-defined areas.

The best introduction to the availability of the 2001 Census is the Census Output Prospectus. It is downloadable via the Census links from the National Statistics website. It describes the OAs, and methods for obtaining data.

In addition to the Prospectus, critical documents include the Output Classification Manual (which describes the data definitions and classifications used in the reporting) and various downloadable manuals that list output tables and area options. Although this documentation will be invaluable to regular and heavy-duty users, great efforts have been made to provide a user-friendly graphical interface, so that many users will find that they can get all they want by navigating the website without downloading supporting documents.

8.4.2 Health

NHS activity data

Two factors have had a major impact on the ability of the NHS to provide data on patient care: first, NPfIT which provides a framework for the development of NHS information systems; second, structural changes, such as the re-structuring of health authorities and regional offices and the increasing role for primary care trusts and the resulting impact on community trusts.

---

[7] The Reason for this is that there is substantial 'list inflation' so that overall, primary care registrations are ~ 6% higher than population estimates.

General practice

There is one officially supported data warehousing scheme, now known as the General Practice Research Database, which is maintained by the Medicines and Health Care Regulator for the Department of Health.

The one comprehensive national resource on general practice activity covers *prescribing*. Details are available from the PPA or the Prescribing Support Unit (PSU).

For several decades, the main national source of data on English general practice have been the surveys that have supported the series of Morbidity Survey in General Practice publications. These data sets are lodged at the data archive.

The triage database systems used by *NHS Direct* are a potentially rich source of information on population morbidity.

There are many examples of local projects successfully approaching general practices and primary care groups and trusts for data on the incidence of specific problems or conditions. There may be no alternative to such local approaches if details on the severity of symptoms or clinical outcomes are required. The most promising conditions are those for which standard care management protocols are established, such as diabetes and asthma.

Some information on *dental care* can be found in the Korner statistics on the Department of Health website. Low level data from the Adult Dental Health Survey and the *Children's Dental Survey* may be available on request from the Department of Health.

The same source should be contacted for access to low-level versions of the 5% sample of dental treatment claims.

The secondary sector

There are two main types of activity data routinely collected and made available for secondary care in the NHS: Hospital Episode Statistics (HES) and Korner data.

Sectors for which information is particularly patchy are the former community health trusts and mental health trusts. Korner returns are the only consistent source of data from these trusts. Several national disease registers are either established or in development, but the cancer registry is probably the only one with national coverage at present.

Access to HES data has much improved with the establishment of an HES site within the Department of Health website and an HES enquiry desk. The HES data dictionary and guide to accessing the data (both can be downloaded from the same source) are good starting points. Many tables of results can be freely downloaded from the website; alternatively, customised requests will be accepted, subject to the usual restrictions to protect patient confidentiality. Most requests can be processed through a low-cost fast-track scheme and free estimates are provided for all requests. Public Health Observations are now providing a HES service to their local public health communities.

The HES and PAS data systems provide the foundation for another major collection of activity statistics, with attached costs. The Healthcare Resource Groups reference data set (available on CD – though access outside the NHS may be restricted) presents patterns of activity for both secondary and some primary care institutions. The PAS/HES material has been processed by a package called 'Grouper' – maintained by the NHS Information Authority (NHSIA). Its aim is to group procedures and episodes of care, within specialities, by the demands they make on healthcare resources. Healthcare providers are then required to estimate the costs of each of these groupings and the reference costs CD reports the age costs by HRG both nationally and by individual trusts. Coverage of all procedures and episodes of care is not yet complete, but the current database is very extensive. The NHSIA website reports progress on extending HRGs beyond the present procedures. The NHS accounting manual (from the Department of Health main site) lists the HRGs that are presently in use for the costings.

8.4.3 Health Surveys

Low level data from most of the main health and health and lifestyle surveys, as well as more general surveys with supplements on health, are lodged with the Data Archive. These include: HSE, the Surveys of Psychiatric Morbidity in Great Britain, GHS and the Omnibus Survey (more details of these can be found in Section 4.2). The SEPHO Lifestyle Toolkit contains online information about lifestyle surveys undertaken.

8.4.4 Social Care

Social services departments in England make a number of annual returns on the services they provide and the numbers of clients. All these data are only available at the level of Local Authorities Responsible for Social Services (LAWRSS) of which there are approximately 150 in England. Some central returns for children's social services now require postcoded data on individual clients and it may be possible to negotiate access to an anonymised ward-based version of this. However, these can be very sensitive data – especially details from the child protection register – and permission may not be granted for ward-level access.

Key Statistics (KS1) is the first and central source for data on personal social services in England.

These are some of the main pieces of information that are available on PSS activity. All are presented by LAWRSS area.

For children:

- Numbers 'being looked after' sub-divided into numbers in different types of care: e.g. residential homes, secure accommodation, fostering and being placed back with families under supervision orders.
- Children with disabilities and special needs.
- Numbers of places in children's homes.

For adults and older adults:

- Numbers of people supported by LAWRSS in residential and nursing homes (also the number of homes and potential places).
- Numbers of people receiving domiciliary care.
- Numbers of people with learning disabilities.

Benefits data (for example on disability) may be a better source of information on the geographical distribution of some of these groups.

8.4.5 Housing

Apart from the Census, very little information on housing is available at sub-local authority level. These are several national surveys, but their samples are too small for sub-LA breakdowns. It is possible to *model* down the survey results, as, for example, in the IMD and Welsh Deprivation Index.

Physical condition of housing

The Census includes questions on amenities such as baths, showers and central heating and the data on numbers of people in the household and the number of rooms occupied are used to compute a measure of overcrowding.

The main sources on the structural condition of housing are two infrequent surveys and local authority returns.

The English House Condition Survey (there are parallels for Wales and Scotland) includes a professional assessment of physical condition and a valuation, as well as an interview with the residents. It is based on a sample of 25,000 dwellings and is repeated every five years. Half of the properties in the 1991 survey were reassessed in 1995 in order to record any changes. The data sets are available from the ODPM.

The ODPM conducts a second national survey, the Survey of English Housing. Here, the emphasis is on the type of accommodation, tenure, the experiences of the household in finding accommodation, moving and their views of the accommodation and the area. The survey is repeated annually and is based on a sample of 20,000 households.

Local authority returns for the HIP give some data on housing stock, vacancies, lettings and homelessness. More specific information is provided by local authority returns on the numbers of unfit dwellings and the reason for their being classified as unfit.

The Housing Needs Index is another LA level data source. It is based on (amongst others) data from the Survey of English Housing, the General Households Survey and the English House Condition Survey.

Housing – tenure

The Survey of English Housing collects information on tenure, but the Census is the main source here. The 1991 Census asked if rented accommodation was furnished or unfurnished. In 2001, this question is only asked in Scotland.

There are several sources relating to particular types of tenure. Housing association statistics (collated by the ODPM) give details of the numbers of lettings and new lettings, also a considerable range of information on the tenants. This information is released for local authority areas.

Local authority housing performance indicators (ODPM) will have some information on tenure.

8.4.6 Employment and Unemployment

Both of the main English sources of unemployment data – the claimant counts and the Labour Force Survey – can be found on the NOMIS website.

Unemployment benefit claimant counts are presented in a number of forms down to ward level. The main options for counts are: counts (age and duration of unemployment), seasonally adjusted counts, unadjusted counts – with rates. The same set of options are available for claimant flows and there is an additional data set of claimant 'off-flows', showing the reason for ceasing to be a claimant in addition to the claimant's age and duration of the most recent claim.

The Labour Force Survey provides an alternative estimate of unemployment independent of the periodic changes in the criteria for claiming unemployment benefit. It is a quarterly sample survey and collects information on personal circumstances and employment status of respondents. The full data sets are lodged with the Data Archive; subsets of recent data are available on-line from NOMIS.

The Annual Employment Survey replaced the annual Census of Employment in late 1995. This survey of approximately 130,000 businesses collects information on the nature of the business, the gender of employees, the types of jobs and whether they are full- or part-time. Data are produced by ward and there is considerable detail on the type of business activity. It is available on-line from NOMIS, but there is a special registration procedure for this data set which requires a statement of intended use.

Other relevant data sets held by NOMIS include details of job centre vacancies, broken down by occupation and industry, but most of these are only available at unitary authority level or higher.

8.4.7 Environment

Local authority returns to the ODPM provide some information here, but there are no national small area data sets.

8.4.8 Crime

Neither of the two main sources of data on crime in England are available at ward level and for this, and related reasons, the compilers of the ODPM reluctantly omitted a crime domain.

The two sources are the annual British Crime Survey and the quarterly returns from police forces to the Home Office. The self-report data from the British Crime Survey can be disaggregated to ACORN type of community within each government region. The annual recorded crime data is available at the basic command unit level (there are about 300 such units per local authority).

Home Office data on notifiable offences recorded by the police are available on the Neighbourhood Statistics Area of the ONS website.

Whenever crime data are presented by electoral ward, the material will have been obtained directly from local police forces. The West Midlands MAIGIS project contains such data on a variety of offences including burglary and car crime for the local area.

The Scottish Area Deprivation Index uses house contents insurance rating at postcode sector as a proxy for crime. Similar data may be available from insurance companies in England.

8.4.9 Education

A limited amount of data on education is provided by the Decennial Census, available from NOMIS. It asks people aged 16 and over to list their educational attainments, and there are boxes to record whether or not each person in the household is a full-time student. The Census also includes a question on professional and vocational qualifications. From 2001, the Census material is available via the main ONS site.

An indirect estimate of those staying in full-time education after the compulsory leaving age can be obtained from child benefit data, which is broken down by the age of child for those aged 16 and over. The Labour Force Survey (from the Data Archive) collects data on adult qualifications.

The DES collects data on educational attainment and absenteeism, but these are nearly always recorded by local educational authority, or educational institution. In the latter case, the catchment area has to be inferred, as there are no published details of the distribution of pupil postcodes. The compilers of the IMD index use GIS techniques to approximate ward maps of primary school catchment areas, but admit that this method is unlikely to be valid for the much larger and complicated secondary school areas. IMD ward-level estimates of *primary school pupils at Key Stage 2* are available on the ONS Neighbourhood Statistics site.

The Universities and Colleges Admissions Service keeps postcoded records of university applicants with details of the outcome of the application. Ward-level university admissions data can be found on the ONS Neighbourhood Statistics site.

8.4.10 Income and Benefits

The New Earnings Survey and Index of Average Earnings are two of the major sources of information on pay and income from work. The former is based on a 1% national sample of employees whose tax is handled via PAYE. Area analyses are available on the NOMIS site. The Index of Average Earnings results are available from the ONS.

Ward-level data on various means-tested and disability-related benefits can be freely downloaded from the ONS Neighbourhood Statistics site.

Income support data is provided by age and household structure in receipt of pensioner, disability or lone parent premiums. Data are also available on numbers of claimants and dependants of claimants. Other counts available at ward level include:

- Family credit claimants.
- Attendance allowance claimants.
- Disability living allowance.
- Jobseeker's allowance.
- Incapacity benefit.
- Severe disablement allowance.

8.4.11 Composite Indicators and Geo-classification Systems

The ONS Classification of local and health authorities, revised for 1999, can be downloaded from the ONS website, or purchased in hard-copy form.

The classification of wards, based on the same system must be purchased from ONS.

Details of the ACORN and SuperProfiles classification systems can be found on-line at www.CACI.co.uk and CLARITAS.co.uk respectively. Descriptions of both are available for free; the databases are for purchase. A licensed version of the higher-level SuperProfile classification may be locally available from the Department of Health.

SECTION 9

DESIGNING SURVEYS TO MEASURE INEQUALITY

9.1 Introduction

Next to the thermometer, probably the most widely used instrument for measuring health status in the U.K. is the following Census question:

> "Do you have any long-term illness, health problem or disability which limits your daily activities or the work you can do?"

The development and use of health status questionnaires has now reached impressive proportions. Broadly speaking there are four classes of instruments:

- Portmanteau questionnaires on health and lifestyle intended for home-based interviews (and sometimes supplemented with physiological measurements).
- General health status questionnaires intended either for use in the general population, or for periodic use in healthcare settings.
- Specialised questionnaires relating to symptoms and various aspects of the life of people with medical conditions.
- Single questions or short batteries of items that are included in non-health questionnaires. These items are often taken from longer health status questionnaires.

The characteristics of the instruments have been reviewed in Section 4. The focus here is on their potential for use in population surveys.

The Portmanteau and general health status questionnaires are routinely used in population surveys.

Specialised questionnaires and short batteries of items are mainly intended for use with patients in medical settings. The dramatic increase in the number of such instruments largely can be explained by the developing interest in obtaining standardised patient reports of the outcomes of care. Despite their clinical focus, some examples of the last two groups are suitable for the mapping of health inequalities with population surveys.

9.2 Surveys and Their Limitations

Regardless of the choice of questionnaire, the validity of the results of a survey will depend to a considerable extent on the sampling strategy and design, details of which can be found in texts on sampling techniques and on questionnaire design. The purpose of this section is to focus on the particularity of surveys for elucidating inequalities in health in your area.

9.2.1 Advantages and Disadvantages

Advantages

- Self-report information can only be obtained from the people concerned, e.g. by asking them (although there are sometimes attemps to solicit proxy information for children and older people).
- Surveys of health provide insights into unmet need and into differences in unmet need between different population groups, because they can collect supporting information on socio-economic characteristics and lifestyle that are rarely kept in medical records.
- With current data systems, surveys may be the best source of information on some types of health service use, especially on aspects of community health services and general practice. This may change as improve.

Disadvantages

However, as a source of information on population morbidity, household or individual surveys have a number of limitations compared with data derived from healthcare administrative systems:

- Survey data (like all data) are subject to a range of errors, including sampling, non-response, coverage and measurement error, which can make results at the small area level statistically unreliable. To avoid this problem, synthetic estimation procedures based on relationships established in the sample have to be used to produce small area estimates [214].
- Surveys cannot collect information that is not related to the characteristics of the respondent (only partial data from the individual's prespective can be collected to measure neighbourhood characteristics such as the extent of community support or social control). It is, however, possible to attach or attribute some geo-demographic information to individual cases if postcoded information on the sample respondents is available.

- Survey assessments of need do not easily translate to potential services or requirements [215]. In some cases, surveys do not even attempt to measure the extent of actual individual need, but simply assess individual service utilisation. These problems could, in principle, be overcome by the use of more sophisticated sampling designs, incorporating some form of independent needs assessment or improved measurement instruments.
- Surveys are generally expensive and time consuming. They cannot anticipate the future; and therefore do not tell us about the characteristics of those who are about to enter hospital, nursing or residential homes.
- It is difficult to obtain valid information for some groups. For example, undertaking a survey to measure children's and families' need for health and family and child care services would be both practically and methodologically difficult. The direct interviewing of children about family and child care problems, within a household or school survey, would pose logistical and ethical problems.
- Unless a survey is accompanied by a medical examination (as in the British Dental Surveys) all evidence on health and health status will be self-reported, complicating any comparisons with the results of surveys with, for example, medically generated incidence data that may use standard-clinical-systems for classifying symptoms and conditions.

In the context of health inequalities, two issues are particularly important:

- Nearly all surveys are of households or of individuals and therefore omit those living – whether permanently or temporarily – in institutions or on the street. Such persons are more likely to be ill, so that one is likely to underestimate overall prevalence. If the purpose is to make comparisons between areas, the problem is compounded because such institutions or the incidence of street living are not distributed equally between areas.
- Non-responses are particularly important in this context because the non-responders may well be the most ill. It is important to compare the sample breakdowns with the Census in terms not only of socio-demographic characteristics but also with the expected percentage reporting a limiting long-term illness (LLTI).

When used for measuring inequalities, results from surveys of health will often be presented as rates, such as the numbers with certain symptoms or poor self-report health per 1000 of the population. Because of the strong associations with age (and often sex) results will frequently need to be standardised by age or by both age and sex (Section 6).

9.2.2 When Not to Do a Survey and the Alternatives

When not to do a survey

Even small surveys can be expensive in time, money and other resources. Surveys that fail to achieve their objectives also incur other costs – they may have inspired false hopes or opened up issues better kept closed. There are often methodological reasons why surveys fail to produce the hoped-for results [216]. Careful design and preliminary checks should help avoid such failures.

Even the most conclusive of surveys is wasted if the report is unread, the proposals rejected or quietly filed. Ensuring that the style, length and presentation of the report is appropriate for the intended readership is one important factor, but if local conditions are unfavourable, it may not be worth starting a survey. Surveys should be avoided if:

- There are insufficient technical and staff resources to conduct the research effectively, especially the analysis and reporting stages.
- The timescale is too tight.
- The data are likely to be inconclusive and no proposals will result.
- The data, or a near equivalent, are already available from official sources or other studies.

Alternatives to surveys

An over-emphasis on the details of survey technique sometimes leads to less formal and less technical research methods being devalued. In academic work, formal methods are used at a late stage in the research, after various sorts of exploratory studies. Obviously, there are times when quantitative data collected by formal methods is essential, but you should be aware of the wide variety of other methods that are available.

Informal data sources

An inequality may become noticeable because of reports in the media, for example, about food poisoning or pollution that has traced back to a particular retailer or factory pollution. In some circumstances, systematic monitoring of the media could substitute for an expensive and potentially inconclusive survey.

Drawbacks of formal methods

Expensive and inconclusive results are not the only reasons for exploring alternatives. One of the great assets of survey research – people's considerable willingness to fill in self-completion questionnaires – hides one of its main drawbacks, that you only get their replies to a series of pre-set questions, not their spontaneous views. Once the fieldwork is over, there is a considerable temptation to forget that what you are confidently describing as your respondents' views are only their replies to your questions, and not necessarily their own interests and priorities. If health service policy has been steered by providers' perceptions and definitions of good practice, should this also hold for consumer research? If one is to emphasise the patients' agenda, how should this be done?

Evidence-based policies need information

There is no such thing as a perfect piece of research. Whilst academic researchers frequently end their report with a plea for further research, they also typically draw attention to how much can be learnt by their approach. The latter is the more appropriate emphasis in this context. The point is to recognise the often fragile information base for present policies, and therefore to realise the scope for improvement. Whilst this does not mean that any information is better than none, it does mean that a wide variety of approaches to collecting information will provide a useful addition to what is known.

9.2.3 *Doing a Survey*

Here we outline the steps one should pay attention to in designing and executing a survey (Table 9.1).

Table 9.1. *Steps to designing and executing a survey*

Step	*Comments*
Specification of Objectives	
Are these clear and potentially answerable by survey?	*If not, return to peer group who suggested survey – DO NOT PROCEED.*
Specify precise aims of survey	*If not, return to objectives*
Propose rough timetable	
Preliminaries	
What do we already know about the situation?	*If enough is known to formulate policy, WHY A SURVEY?*
Look at reports of similar studies	
Pre-piloting, finding out which kinds of questions will be appropriate	*If this is not done, statistics will not save you*
Draw up a sampling plan	
Will any of the analysis require technical input?	

(*Continued*)

Table 9.1. *(Continued)*

Step	*Comments*
Survey design to include:	
whether interview or self-completion;	
sampling plan and rough size of sample (this might be as simple as a choice of clinics and a number of days);	
length and style of questionnaires;	
proposed staff and training;	
plan for fieldwork (crucially proposed dates, times and proposed location of staff);	
preparations for coding, data entry;	*If you will need statistical/technical advice get it now*
plan for analysis;	
rough timetable for survey.	
Seeking agreement on sampling points from floor management	
Re-examine design of survey for technical inputs	
Questionnaire Design	
Produce first draft of questionnaire. Circulate to interested parties. Try it on friends.	*Remember the potential respondents are at best patient, probably long-suffering, and may not read or speak English fluently. Do not make it worse by asking them to answer an incomprehensible question*
Piloting, trying out the draft questionnaire on small number of the potential respondents	*If it looks as if you would not get the answers you need, DO NOT PROCEED*
Analyse the responses from the pilot	
Final approval from colleagues	*Return to examine aims of research and whether design is appropriate*
Setting up	
Choosing staff for interviewing	*Good interviewers are rare; they need to be insistent, but extremely pleasant with it*
Choosing staff for clerical work	*Although much of work is clerical, accuracy is obviously very important*
Finalise fieldwork plan (dates, times and location of staff)	
Execution	
Data Collection	*Regular spot visits by you to see how things are going*
Running record of progress	*Compare with sampling plan*
Coding and data entry	*If possible, arrange for checking*
Analysis	*Refer repeatedly to original aims of survey*
Report writing	
Discuss proposed draft with peer group and management	
Formal report for action	
Monitor effectiveness	

9.3 Assuming You Have Decided on a Survey

9.3.1 Getting Your Objectives Clear: What Do You Want to Find Out?

Information is only useful when your objectives are clear. Many studies fail to reach tangible conclusions simply because they fail to define their aims beyond "wanting to find out about the distribution of limiting long-standing illness". It is often difficult to reach policy relevant conclusions with a general purpose questionnaire.

What will be the nature of your results?

You should realise that, with most surveys, the results are broadly predictable. They are unlikely to tell you anything new, only to provide you with quantitative estimates of the relative importance of the various factors. Indeed, the most likely surprises are that certain factors are NOT as important as you thought they were.

The need for comparisons

Secondly, very little can be done with absolute percentages. Suppose you find limiting long-term illness levels in your area is between 15 and 20%, does this mean things are going well or badly? Answering inequality-type questions requires comparative data. This could come from the same study, when you might be comparing results from several different units, or from previous studies done either in your area or elsewhere.

The need for comparisons raises three further points:

- There should be greater standardisation in the questions asked. There are a large number of examples of how different dimensions of inequality can be measured (Section 2), and a wide range of scales have been developed for measuring different aspects of health (Section 3).
- It is difficult to make effective comparisons with results from weak questions, e.g. when the wording tends to get the same response from most informants.
- Even if percentage differences show that some groups report more limiting long-term illness than others, they do not tell you causation or etiology.

Making recommendations based on your survey

The potential effectiveness of a survey should be tested by running a trial analysis on your pilot data and checking that it is capable of informing the sort of recommendations you want. Do not forget to record open-ended comments as these are often very useful in illustrating the discussion of your findings.

9.3.2 Research and Academic Criteria

How important is it to observe the technical criteria, what the 'research methodologist' says you should do? There is a tendency for non-academic authors to distance themselves from 'research'.

The notion that one set of criteria applies to health service surveys and another for academic research is unsound. Health service surveys may pay more attention to questions of effectiveness, and may be more descriptive than hypothesis testing but, they still benefit from good design. A survey which has only a 30% response rate will have expended considerable resources trying unsuccessfully to reach the other 70%. It will have no way of telling whether policy based on the views of that particular minority is likely to be acceptable to the other 70%, though one suspects that with such a low response rate, certain groups will be systematically under-represented. One should automatically be suspicious of a questionnaire giving such low response rates; for example, were the questions incoherent or irrelevant such that many respondents gave up?

There are some very technical forms of data analysis and accuracy estimation that are unlikely to be relevant for many surveys, but the vast majority of methodological criteria, are really just ways of ensuring conclusive and cost-effective surveys.

9.3.3 Research Aims

Surveys will normally have one or more of the following purposes:

- *Explanatory studies.* These would usually be the first stage of any research where one is uncertain of the issues. They can include literature searches, and interviews with 'experts' and others in the area. Exploratory studies may either be a preliminary to developing more formal methods, such as a pre-coded questionnaire, or may be worthwhile exercises in themselves in developing knowledge of a little known area.
- *Descriptive studies.* These are the type most often used in patient-feedback studies. Their aim is usually to collect data, which can influence or evaluate policy. Although descriptive, they should still have well-defined objectives, e.g. one should be precisely sure what range of data is needed and how it might lead to specific recommendations.
- *Hypothesis testing surveys.* These are widely used in socio-medical research. A typical study might aim to explore links between dietary patterns and a particular medical condition. They differ in two main respects from the descriptive model. First, their sampling strategy will require some sort of control group. Second, their analysis is unlikely to stop at basic frequency counts and cross-tabulations, and will include various forms of multi-variate analyses. Though less

common than descriptive studies, hypothesis testing is also used in patient-feedback research, especially when the project sets out to test the effects of a specific change.

- *Other motives*. Finally, there are a variety of studies for which data collection is a secondary aim. Their intentions differ, but are usually either some form of public relations, or some attempt to demonstrate research activity.

9.4 Different Types of Survey

Cross-sectional surveys or 'snapshot' approach is the most common, but surveys of health may often benefit from other designs. They are the most common form of feedback research, though one also finds examples of panel, quasi-panel and standing-panel models.

9.4.1 Cross-Sectional Studies Versus Longitudinal Surveys

Cross-Sectional Surveys are simply surveys conducted at a single point in time. If they aim to be explanatory or test some hypothesis, they require a control group. If they are mainly descriptive, a control may not be necessary. A well-designed cross-sectional study can be as valid or 'scientific' as a longitudinal study.

At the same time, there are situations in which one would have much more confidence in inferences based on repeated observations over time on a set of variables for the set of persons belonging to the survey. An important constraint on the design of a longitudinal survey is the specification of the purposes the survey is to serve and to identify their operational and budget constraints. Choosing the most appropriate survey design requires assessing the benefits of the different sorts of information provided and the different costs required to derive them.

9.4.2 Obtaining Longitudinal Data through Health Surveys

There are four main ways of deriving these repeated observations on the same people through a survey:

- *Retrospective*: wherein respondents are typically interviewed only once and they are asked about the past.
- *Record linkage*: in which responses from the sample respondents are linked to their health service records.
- *Quasi-panel surveys*: in which the responses from a before group *are compared* with those of an after group.
- *Panel (or longitudinal) surveys*: wherein the same sample of persons (a 'panel') is followed over time, and data are collected from a sequence of interviews ('waves').

Retrospective surveys

In retrospective surveys, respondents are typically interviewed only once and they are asked about the past as well as the present in order to provide two (or more) observations on the same person. The advantages of this method are its simplicity and cheapness (because there is only a single interview: respondents do not have to be tracked), and the immediate availability of longitudinal information (since one does not have to wait for a second interview to measure change). The principal disadvantages are that information about the past is typically dependent on respondents' recall of events, and the accuracy of this is questionable for some variables of policy interest. People are unlikely, for example, to remember very well their income beyond the immediate past,[8] or may do so in a biased way. On the other hand, the dates of significant, low frequency, lifetime events such as getting married or divorced, having a child, or changes in one's main job, are more likely to be remembered with reasonable accuracy. These latter events have been the focus of retrospective social surveys.

Record linkages

Another important approach is to link together information from diverse sources, for example, from respondents and from their health service records. The Data Protection Act, however, often precludes this sort of linkage. Even when it is acceptable, it is rather difficult because of the different ways in which the crucial identification variables have been constructed in the different sources.

Nevertheless, where it is possible, often very important information can be obtained. A study carried out by the National Primary Care Research and Development Centre interviewed respondents about their visits to surgery and asked for permission to approach their GPs for access to their records. The study showed that there were significant discrepancies in the respondents' recall of diagnosis and what had been recorded in their General Practitioners' files.

Quasi-panel surveys

The presumption here is that the current before group can be compared to a current after group as if they were identical. Though not normally providing valid comparisons, and therefore not recommended, the quasi-panel method is frequently used. In the health survey context, we frequently compare the results, for example, of the GHS across several years without paying as much attention as we should to issues of comparability of the samples in different years.

---

[8] One estimate is that the recall of small items of household expenditure 'decays' by nearly 3% a day!

Panel surveys

Panel surveys are ones in which a sample of informants ('the panel') are contacted more than once to find if they, their experiences and opinions, have changed over time. Perhaps, the most famous British panel studies are the birth cohort studies conducted on large samples of all children born in single weeks in 1946, 1958 and 1970.

The simplest panel design interviews an individual both before and after a course of treatment. There are many possible variations, but the main distinction is between surveys comprising a single panel of indefinite life, and surveys comprising multiple overlapping panels of fixed life, also known as rotating panel surveys. A second distinction refers to the sampling unit and the population that the survey aims to represent – whether the focus is entirely at the individual level, or on individuals within their household context. This distinction helps define the rules about who comprises the panel beyond the initial sample: which people in the original panel are followed over time, and how (if at all) new panel members might replenish survey numbers. The issue is quite complex (Appendix to Section 9). A third distinction refers to the types of longitudinal information collected by the panel survey, in particular, the extent to which data are collected about life prior to the first interview wave and about life between waves.

9.5 Summary

Advantages

- You can only get self-report information from people by asking them.
- Surveys can provide insights into unmet need.
- With current data systems, surveys may be the best source of information on some types of health service use.

Disadvantages

- Survey data (like all data) are subject to a range of errors, including sampling, non-response, coverage and measurement error.
- Surveys can only collect information related to the characteristics of the respondent.
- Survey assessments do not easily translate to potential services or requirements.
- Surveys are expensive and time consuming.
- It is difficult to obtain valid information for some groups.
- Nearly all evidence on health and health status will be self-reported, complicating any comparisons with the results of surveys with medically generated incidence data.

In the context of health inequalities, there are two other issues that must be remembered:

- Nearly all surveys are of households, and therefore omit those living in institutions or on the street.
- The importance of accounting for non-responses because the non-responders may well be the most ill.

Main types of design

- Cross-sectional surveys.
- Retrospective surveys.
- Record linkage surveys.
- Quasi-panel surveys.
- True panel surveys.

SECTION 10

INEQUALITIES AND METHODS OF MEASUREMENT

This section takes a more detailed and technical look at the way in which inequality can be measured, the properties of different indexes and their measurement; various approaches to summarising inequality; and how one might measure inequalities in health over time.

10.1 Introduction

This section will be of use mainly to practitioners who are more familiar with statistical concepts and who may be more interested in the theoretical basis for the development and evaluation of measures of inequality. As such, it may be used together with the practical sections giving guidance on how to apply or develop indexes and/or surveys on poverty, deprivation, health, disease and lifestyles (see Sections 3–6 and 9).

The section opens with a short introduction to some of the main issues in measuring inequalities (repeated from Section 1). Section 10.3 then considers some properties of both indexes and methods of measurement that may be more appropriate to specific applications. Section 10.4 examines different techniques for detecting and analysing inequality. Section 10.5 highlights some issues in trying to measure (changes in) inequality over time.

10.2 Context

Two questions are central to the measurement of inequality – what is meant by inequality and how to measure it.

What is meant by inequality

Three concepts are frequently used:

- Differences or variations in health (or income) between groups.
- Inequalities in health(or income).
- Inequities or the unfairness of differences.

Throughout, the term 'variations' is reserved for purely statistical usage and inequalities is used in its descriptive sense. Although the fairness of the differences in health between SEGs is not discussed here, the purpose of measuring inequalities is because they point to *likely* inequities.

> Kunst and Mackenbach use the following working definition of health inequalities: "Differences in the prevalence or incidence of health problems between individual people of higher and lower socio-economic status" (1995)

It should be emphasised that although the definition refers to individuals, *the crucial characteristic is their membership of an SEG*. Whilst differences between individuals may well be interesting in themselves, they are only meaningful in terms of inequalities or inequities if those differences are linked to socio-economic status or some other dimension of differentiation (e.g. ethnicity or religion).

How to measure inequality

Most measurement of health inequality involves the use of indicators or indexes to measure health, but it also requires decisions on what groups or areas to compare and what is the most appropriate form of analysis for the question being investigated.

In short, devising a method for measuring inequalities requires answers to three questions:

- What is the comparator, are inequalities to be measured between:
  Groups or populations of small areas (Section 2).
  Countries or populations to which different socio-economic classification have been applied (Sections 2 and 10).
  Similar groups or populations over time (Section 10).
- What type of inequality is of interest:
  Relative or absolute inequality (Sections 10 and 11).
  Risk based versus outcome based measure (Section 10).
- What is the intended use for index of inequality:
  To monitor the impact of policies and practices (often governmental policies and practices) on specific populations (Sections 10 and 11).
  To compile league tables (Sections 10 and 11).

10.3 Properties of Indexes and Measurements

When measuring inequality, the indexes and measurements will require different properties for different applications. We have examined the range of possible axes of differentiation (Section 2) and the adequacy of data from routine sources or from surveys for measuring health (Sections 3 and 4, respectively). We have discussed the technical properties of indexes in general (Section 8). In this section we discuss the technical properties of indexes of inequality. We consider below: simplicity, absolute or relative measures, and measurement of effect or of total impact.

Simplicity

Policy makers tend to ask for simple measures that can be readily understood, for example death as a measure of health, and employment status as a measure of socio-economic position. The problem with simple measures is that they may only partially capture what one is interested in. Death is a consequence of poor health, but is not the same; employment status is a very 'thin' description of inequality. Researchers and statisticians should try to compare results of analyses based on simple measures with the results of analyses using more sophisticated summary measures of the various components of the particular phenomenon. It is of course, preferable if the components of measures are easily understandable and logically linked to what is being measured.

Absolute or relative terms

The usual presentation of inequalities, is in *relative* terms, for example, the mortality rates of the lowest SEGs as a ratio to that of the highest SEG. The alternate presentation is in *absolute* terms for example, the differences between the mortality of the highest and the lowest SEG.

Both of these are important, and probably should be used in combination. It is common to assess the importance of difference in relative rather than absolute terms; however, a 50% higher rate of a rare health problem may be much less important to public health than a 10% higher rate of a frequent health problem. Presentation of the absolute difference would make this clear.

Measures of effect and measures of total impact

The crucial distinction here is between the measure of the effect of changes in socio-economic status on health status, compared to a measure of total impact on the health of the whole population, taking into account the distribution of socio-economic characteristics within the population.

Of course, the size of SEGs makes a difference and with changes in the occupational structure, the groups change, so that similar segments of the population are not being compared.

Where summary measures are used, it is preferable if the components of the measures are easily understandable and linked to what is being measured.

Statistical properties of indexes

Some aspects of the properties of indexes' domains have already been discussed in Sections 2 and 4 on measures of health and Sections 5 and 6 on measures of deprivation. Section 7 provides a more detailed account of the statistical characteristics of indexes, particularly tests for reliability and validity. Notions of reliability and validity, especially the latter, can be interpreted in many ways, and particular interpretations might be relevant to particular applications, e.g. an instrument that was valid or reliable for one purpose, might not be for another.

Different methods make different demands on their data. It may be that an instrument that generates data suitable for making summaries of overall inequality between individuals is not suitable for making comparisons between groups. Or it may be that a policy-orientated application encourages the use of simple measures, but such measures may not have the responsiveness to detect likely levels of inequalities.

10.4 Approaches to Summarising Inequality

10.4.1 Simple Inequality Measures

The first discussions on inequalities in health relied on relatively simple comparisons between specific groups, for example, a comparison between the death rates of Social Classes I and II compared to the death rates in Social Classes IV and V. These are still used by many, but they do have problems. In particular, because they focus on particular groups, such comparisons ignore some of the information about the distribution of health between all the members of the population. In this section, we discuss the advantages and disadvantages of indexes that attempt to summarise the way in which health is distributed across the *whole* population.

Measures that compare two groups

Range

This involves comparing the experiences of the top and bottom SEGs. The comparison is commonly presented as the ratio of one extreme value to the other.

It is of course, crucial to know what aspect of health is being compared between the two groups. Clearly, disparities in the risk of early death are important, and, in a situation where many die early, it may well be the only dimension of 'health' worth examining. But, when more people are living

Table 10.1. *Age-specific annual mortality rates per 100,000 between 25 and 64 and survivors at age 65 and 85 (1960 and 1981)*

	Annual mortality rate per 100,000				*% of survivors of a cohort age 65 with these death rates*	*Proportion of population age 85+*
	25–34	*35–44*	*45–54*	*55–64*		
1960						
Men	112	241	717	2140	73	0.2
Women	73	173	435	1060	84	0.6
1981						
Men	88	179	600	1732	77	0.5
Women	51	124	374	929	86	1.6

beyond 65, the variation in age at death among those over 65 will decrease, so that 'inequalities in health' – measured by differences between the average age at death for different social groups – will also decrease.

One could continue to argue that early deaths are so important that the conventional measure is to be preferred, but it needs to be understood that it refers to only a small proportion of deaths. Inequalities in death are not the only possible focus. If one looks at inequalities in survivorship beyond 65, one gets rather a different picture (Table 10.1). Whilst the death rates for men are always at least 39% higher than those for women in each age group, the proportion of women who survive beyond 65 is only 12% larger. Similarly whilst inequalities in survivorship between social classes persist, there has been only a small reduction from 15% to 12% in the difference between the percentage *not* surviving to 75, and a halving of the percentage difference in those not surviving to 85 (Table 10.2).

The statistical defects of focussing only on the differences between extreme groups should be obvious. First, what goes on in intermediate groups is ignored. For example, the gap between top and bottom groups might remain unchanged, but the extent of inequality between the intermediate groups might well be diminishing (or increasing). The second problem with the range is that it takes no account of the size of the groups being compared. In one of the favourite comparisons between social

Table 10.2. *Social class and survival beyond 65. England and Wales*

	Percentage not survived to 75 years			*Percentage survival to 85 years*		
	1951	*1971*	*1981*	*1951*	*1971*	*1981*
Manual	55.5	56.8	60.7	11.5	13.0	16.2
Non-manual	63.7	63.0	67.9	20.8	21.0	22.7

classes, this is crucial as the size of these groups vary substantially over time. As Illsley [217] put it, "if we wished to compare two countries over time, our first step would be to check the boundaries".

The impact of this on comparisons of death rates has been examined by Carr-Hill [218]. Whilst one may be more interested in comparisons of morbidity rates than in the comparison of death rates between geographical areas, the general point about the potential impact of the changes in composition of populations in, for example, communities on the validity of comparison over time, is very important.

Comparing groups of equal size

The problem with all discrete classifications, is that the population distribution changes in both size and significance over time. The only real solution to this problem, is to compare the bottom 10% (or 20%) with the top 10% (or 20%) at different points in time. Clearly the 'bottom' and 'top' deciles or quintiles have to be defined in terms of some socio-economic criterion. The ideal characteristic would be continuous such as income. If a continuous variable is not available, then members of the population have to be classified and ranked in terms of categorical criteria such as education, occupation or geographical area.

10.4.2 More Complicated Measures

Because of the problems with discrete classifications, increasing numbers of researchers have developed measures based on continuous variables.

The Lorenz curve and the Gini coefficient

One of the proposed 'solutions' has been to examine an aggregate measure of inequalities between individuals such as the Gini coefficient, as is done in assessing inequalities in the distribution of income and wealth [219]. Le Grand [219] proposed comparing global measures of dispersion between individuals, not between strata. The coefficient he used is based on the Lorenz curve.

Lorenz curve

The 'pure' Lorenz curve is a graphical representation showing the degree of inequality of a frequency distribution in which the cumulative percentage of the variable under study (e.g. morbidity or mortality) is plotted on the Y-axis against the cumulative percentage of the population ordered/ranked (along the X-axis) according to the variable under study. A straight line rising at an angle of 45° from the origin on the graph will indicate perfect equality; for instance, if the 10% with the lowest incomes account for 10% of the deaths, 20% with the lowest incomes account for 20% of the deaths and so on.

If, however, the distribution is not precisely egalitarian then the curve will be above or below the diagonal. The greater the distance of the curve from the diagonal line, the greater the inequality. When the variable considered is beneficial to the population, for example, access to healthy lifestyles, the curve is found below the diagonal line. In contrast, when the variable is prejudicial, for example deaths, it is found above the line. So, where there is a larger rate of deaths among men with lower incomes and a smaller rate of deaths among those with higher incomes, the distribution is unequal. When such a distribution is plotted, a curve will be traced above the 45° line and the degree of curvature will be greater, the greater the inequality (Figure 10.1).

This line is the Lorenz curve and can be expressed mathematically. The Gini coefficient ranges from 0 to 1 (0 representing perfect equality and 1 total inequality). It corresponds to twice the area between the Lorenz curve and the diagonal (Figure 10.1).

Although the level of inequalities is reflected in the value of the Gini coefficient itself, the interpretation of the coefficient is usually done in comparative terms, by contrasting the calculated value to that of other geographic units, population groups, etc. Again, a coefficient of 0.2 will represent a lower level of inequality than a coefficient of 0.4. The cumulative proportions of both variables (the 'health' variables and the SEG variables) can also be read directly from the graphical representation of the Lorenz curve.

Figure 10.1. *Lorenz curves. Notes: A = line of equality; B = Country 1; C = Country 2; D = line of absolute inequality.*

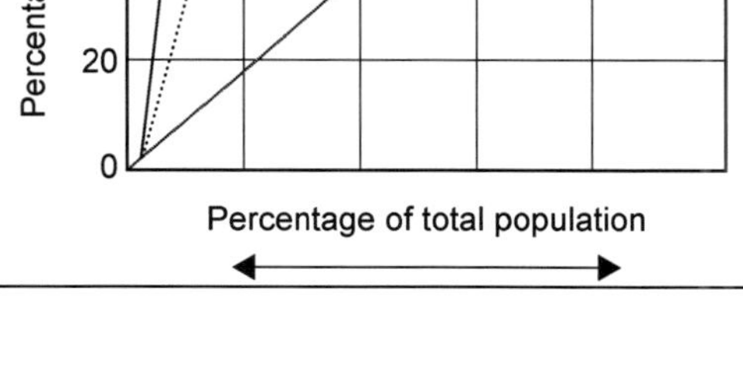

There are different methods to calculate the Gini coefficient. One example, provided by Brown, to calculate the Gini coefficient and prepare a graph demonstrating inequalities between geographic units, the Lorenz curve [220]:

1. Sort the geographic units by the health variable (e.g. infant mortality rate) from the worst situation (highest rate), to the best situation (lowest rate).
2. Calculate the number of infant deaths for each geographic unit.
3. Calculate what proportion of the total of all infant deaths and what proportion of the total of all live births is observed in each geographical unit.
4. Calculate the cumulative proportion of each of the two variables.
5. Calculate the Gini coefficient using the formula.
6. Graph the curve using the *X* axis for the proportion of the cumulative population (live births) and the *Y* axis for the proportion of cumulative health variable observations (infant deaths).

The Lorenz curve reflects the experiences of all the persons rather than only those in specific groups, and the size of this dispersion may well be crucial in assessing the overall importance of the issue. For example, deaths from bronchitis, influenza, pneumonia and respiratory tuberculosis, which used to be one of the major public health issues during the first half of this century, have now fallen to a very low level overall, even though their distribution is very unequal. Changes in the size of the dispersion (or the gap) do influence our assessments about inequality, but so does the overall level or trend of the problem.

Regardless of the magnitude, the dispersion between individuals cannot be the basis for assessing the inequity of a distribution. This is because dispersion per se cannot be a basis for deciding whether or not a characteristic is unequally distributed in social terms. The absence of a stratifying variable means that the Gini coefficient is addressing a different question from that being addressed in the bulk of the literature-to what extent are there inequalities in health that are systematically related to socio-economic status? This is because a change in the distribution of health where a sick person gets less sick and a healthy person gets less well so that they are both near the mean level of health is registered as a reduction in inequality irrespective of the socio-economic status of the persons concerned. Inequality measured by the Gini coefficient would still fall even if the sick person getting healthier were rich and the healthy person getting sicker were poor.

Most authors therefore argue that measuring health inequality across individuals without taking into account any dimension of (socio-economic) differentiation is not interesting:

> "the main problem is that such a measure (of individual inequality) answers a different – possibly rather uninteresting – question about generalised

variability within a society distinct from systematic variability based on social stratification within society" [221].

Nevertheless, it should be noted that the measures of health inequality proposed by Murray et al. [222] as part of the recent WHO ranking of health systems are of the same type.

The 'pseudo' Lorenz curve and the index of dissimilarity

The problem is circumvented by constructing a 'pseudo' Lorenz curve based on the grouped data, where the groups are occupational classes (or could be classes grouped according to any other socio-economic criterion). The occupational classes are grouped by their health status and then the 'Lorenz' curve graphs the cumulative percentage of the population in their occupational class groups, against the cumulative percentage of death. Although not usually a problem – because the classes are grouped according to their health status – the approach cannot differentiate between a situation when the sickest SEG is made up of rich people versus poor people.

The Index of Dissimilarity (ID) is developed from this curve. It is based on the notion that under complete equality, everyone's share of health (S_{H}) would be equal to their population share (S_{P}). Suppose there are five SEGs S_1, S_2, S_3, S_4, S_5. Then the ID is calculated as half the sum of the absolute values of the differences:

$$\mathrm{ID} = \frac{1}{2}[(S_{1\mathrm{h}} - S_{1\mathrm{p}}) + (S_{2\mathrm{h}} - S_{2\mathrm{p}}) + (S_{3\mathrm{h}} - S_{3\mathrm{p}}) + (S_{4\mathrm{h}} - S_{4\mathrm{p}}) + (S_{5\mathrm{h}} - S_{5\mathrm{p}})]$$

The problem is that the ID, although apparently incorporating a socio-economic dimension, is actually insensitive to the socio-economic dimension of inequalities in health, like the 'pure' Lorenz curve. What matters in the ID is simply how each SEG's share of the population's health compares with its share of population, and not how this disparity compares with a group's socio-economic status.

The Gini coefficient, and similar indexes, can be used correctly in this context – for such a measure can be used to summarise the differences between the levels and/or rates in each population stratum adjusting, where appropriate, for the different sizes of the strata. Note this is a different interpretation of the Gini coefficient to that given above. Preston et al. [223] used the Gini coefficient to assess trends over time, and showed how other coefficients – the ID and an index derived from the regression of age standardised class death rates with the proportions of the population in each social class – gave similar results.

The Slopes and Relative Index of Inequality

Both these indexes, in contrast, are based on the socio-economic dimension to inequalities in health. Classes or groups are ranked by their socio-economic status and these graphical presentations display both their mean health status (represented by the height of the bar) and their share of the population (represented by the width of the bar). The Slope Index of Inequality (SII) is then defined as the slope of the regression line showing the relationship between a class or group's health status and its rank in socio-economic terms. It can be interpreted as the *absolute* effect on average health of moving up one unit in the socio-economic scale.

Because the data are grouped, one cannot equate a one unit change to a shift of one rank with socio-economic scale. This means that the calculation of the SII is not entirely straightforward, requiring the use of weighted least squares. This can be done by summing Ordinary Least Squares on the following equation:

$$h_j\sqrt{n_j} = \alpha\sqrt{n_j} + \beta\chi_j\sqrt{n_j} + u_j$$

where h_j is the health score in class j, n_j is the size of class j, χ_j, is the relative rank of class j.

SII avoids the defects of the range measure; it reflects the experience of the entire population and it is sensitive to the distribution of the population across SEGs.

Note that, if everyone's health improves, as over the past two centuries, then the index can change in value, even though it will be unclear whether one would want to say inequality had changed. Thus, if everyone were sick on half as many days per year as before, then the value of the index would double because the absolute differences have widened. Because this makes comparisons over time difficult, Pamuk [224] proposed dividing the SII by the mean level of health and this is called the Relative Index of Inequality (RII).

The Concentration Index

This index is based on a curve. It is superficially similar to the Lorenz curve, but avoids its problems because people are ranked – as with the SII and the RII – by their socio-economic status and not by their health. The curve plots the cumulative proportions of the population (beginning with the most disadvantaged and ending with the least disadvantaged) against the cumulative proportion of health. The Concentration Index is then calculated in the same way as the Gini coefficient, but it varies between -1 and $+1$. The values are negative when the curve is above the diagonal and positive when they are under the diagonal. If the order resulting from sorting by the socio-economic and health variables are the same, the Concentration Index will have the same absolute value as the Gini coefficient.

If health is equally distributed, the Concentration curve will coincide with the diagonal. If poor health is concentrated in lower SEGs, the Concentration curve lies below the diagonal.

The Health Concentration Index – usually denoted by *C* – is defined as twice the area between the concentration curve and the diagonal.

The same approach can be used for assessing inequalities in ill health, and is, perhaps, easier to understand in this context. The Illness Concentration Index is positive when the Concentration curve lies below the diagonal (illness is concentrated amongst the higher SEGs) and negative when it lies above the diagonal (illness is concentrated among lower SEGs).

The Concentration Index refers to cumulative *proportions* of health and so is insensitive to changes in the mean level of health. It can be generated by graphing the cumulative percentage of the population (along the X-axis) against the cumulative *amount* of health (along the Y-axis). The *Generalised Concentration Index* is then defined as twice the area between the generalised concentration curve and the diagonals.

10.5 Measuring Inequalities in Health Over Time

Understandably, there is considerable interest in measuring in inequalities in health over time. This poses particular problems of interpretation and validity if there is the likelihood of the measure having changed its meaning over the period in question.

For this reason, measuring inequalities in morbidity and making comparisons over time are even more difficult than making comparisons between SMRs. This is basically because health means different things to different people, and meanings change over time.

10.6 Summary and Conclusions: Choosing between the Measures

These various indexes and methods of measurement can be summarised in terms of the properties that we outlined in the beginning: simplicity, whether or not one is interested in absolute or relative measures, and measurement of effect or of total impact. The results of this comparison are shown in Table 10.3. Some of the similarities in the properties are unexpected, as it can be shown that the Concentration Index and the RII are related, as are the Generalised Concentration Index and the SII.

Table 10.3. *Characteristics of indexes for analysing inequality*

Degree of complexity	*Indexes of effect*	*Indexes of total impact comparison with*	
		Healthiest	*Average*
Simpler	Rate ratio of lowest versus highest group	Population-attributable risk (%)	Index of Dissimilarity (%)
	Rate difference of lowest versus highest group	Population attributable risk (N)	Index of Dissimilarity (N)
More complex	Regression-based index of relative effect	Regression-based population attributable risk (%)	Relative Index of Inequality
	Regression-based index of absolute effect	Regression-based population attributable risk (absolute version)	Slope Index of Inequality

SECTION 11

CONTEXT, HISTORY AND THEORY

11.1 Introduction

The measurement of inequality does not take place in isolation; in many countries, there are established bodies of research. There is a sense of what are key questions from different academic and political perspectives, and theories on the nature of inequality and its causes.

It is hard to ignore this context when investigating inequalities and important to assess the extent to which existing approaches and prior results are influencing the work in hand. In this section, we introduce some theories on investigating inequality in the U.K., highlighting ways in which the choice of approach may influence the results.

11.2 Context

The existence and persistence of inequalities in health has been a matter of public record and commentary in the U.K. for a very long time, since the Registrar General's Social Class Classification was designed for use with the 1911 Census, to help search for an explanation for inequalities in death rates [1].

Discussion on the issue was re-ignited in 1980 by the partial suppression by the Conservative Government of the report on inequalities in health commissioned under the previous Labour Government (the Black Report). Scholars in other European countries quickly documented similar disparities and by 1987 the European region of the WHO adopted the reduction of 25% in health inequalities as the first target of its 'Health for All' by the Year 2000 programme.

More recent data from the ONS longitudinal study including figures for 1997–1999 shows that the gap between males in Social Class I (professionals) and males in Social Class V (manual workers) has narrowed since 1992–1996. Life expectancy for males in Social Class V has risen at a faster rate than life expectancy for Social Class I males. Looking at the gradient, it seems as though the difference between I and V has reverted to how it was in the 1970s and 1980s, although with a higher average life expectancy, and that the figures in the early 1990s were the ones that were out of step with the trend.

Distinguishing between methods and results

Although inequality may be readily recognised, the wide range of possible measures both of the dimension of (socio-economic) differentiation and of health itself, means that it is not easy to reach agreement over the level of inequality. Indeed, there may be a confusion of methods of measurement with analysis of the extent of inequalities, or of their causes themselves. Different methods of measurement, or different approaches to monitoring lead to different results. Many researchers who favour a particular conclusion or cause have therefore tended to privilege the method which leads to that conclusion.

Instead, an examination of methods and of their technical properties should be treated as a topic distinct from the findings of empirical analyses using those methods. However, the distinction cannot always be maintained:

- Any methods of summarising distributions of necessity imposes weights on different parts of the distribution and those weights can be disputed. Compare, for example, a ratio of rates at the top and bottom, with a measure like the Gini coefficient.
- The repeated use of one dimension for displaying differences tends to imply causality. For example, the persistent breakdown by age, race, and sex in the first U.S. social indicators implies that race was a causal factor leading to the observed differences.
- Some methods of measurement are best applied at an individual level and others at an area level, which can imply or constrain discussion of causation. For example, the discussion around Le Grand's [219] argument for the comparison of global measures of dispersion between individuals not between strata.

Clearly, issues like these cannot be ignored, but given the independent existence of the science of measurement, with a wide range of technical properties of measures and methods which are independent of the results and of their interpretation, it is important to respect scientific rigour in any such study undertaken.

11.3 The Principal Theoretical Frameworks for Approaching Inequalities

Although there has been no attempt in this handbook to explain the level and/or trends in inequalities in British Society, it is important to understand the existing theoretical interpretative framework within which these issues that are usually discussed. Much has now been published within the framework of the original four-fold choice of explanation in the Black Report. They proposed four kinds of explanation: the *artefactuality* of comparing Registrar General Social Class distributions over time, the role of *social-selection* in producing the observed distributions, the *material and structural conditions affecting health*, and the influence of different sub-cultural *patterns of health-related behaviour*. Although, with hindsight, this model now seems hardly ideal, it has been such common currency that it is hard to avoid making it the basis of any discussion.

This section therefore focuses mainly on the four approaches identified in the Black Report (Sections 11.3.1–11.3.4), but it also includes a discussion of the ideas behind presentations of inequalities in avoidable death (Section 11.3.5) and comparisons of income inequalities and health inequalities (Section 11.3.6).

The Original four-fold model

11.3.1 Artefactuality

The Working Group on Inequalities in Health (WGIH) considered what it called the *artefact* issue – the reliability of the measurement tool itself, which can affect the validity of an SMR at a point in time.

The numerator–denominator bias

The numerator is based on the occupational distribution among those who die during the period considered. The denominator is based on the occupational distribution at the most recent Census.

Indeed, an earlier Decennial Supplement on Occupational Mortality (OPCS, 1986) advised against the comparison of SMRs over time for this reason. They illustrated their argument for Social Class V, focussing on labourers and unskilled workers not elsewhere classified (nec). They present the comparison of SMRs calculated at the two Censuses apparently showing how the SMRs for Social Class V had increased substantially, but showing that this was because of the contribution of those not elsewhere classified (Table 11.1). If those groups are excluded the rates for Social Class V fall substantially. They suggested that, “the most likely explanation is that the power of the Census to classify persons to more specific occupations improved to a greater extent than death registration over the period”. But an estimate from the Longitudinal Study (a cohort of approximately 1% of the population followed up from Census to Census with replacement) over the same period does not show these dramatic differences; so that can be only part of the explanation.

These 'technical' difficulties are serious and cannot be dismissed. There is, perhaps, a more damning criticism of using the RG Social Class Classification in this context; it is simply that the occupational mortality tables give peculiar results.

Table 11.1. *Mortality for labourers and unskilled workers and Social Class V England and Wales (1970–1972, 1979–1980, and 1982–1983)*

	Standardised mortality ratio (all men = 100)		
Occupation/class	*1970–1972*	*1979–1980 1982–1983**	*1971–1981*
Labourers and unskilled workers nec-other (114,160.8)	201	355	129
Labourers and unskilled workers nec-total (XVIII, 160)	141	242	124
Social class V	137	163	124
Social class V excluding labourers and unskilled workers nec total	106	73	124

Note: nec, not elsewhere classified.
Source: OPCS [114].

Demographic shifts in the social classes

The more serious contention is simply that the size of the RG Social Classes has changed over time and that this invalidates any over-time comparisons between the death rates of different RG Social Classes. Despite assertions that "the change in the distribution of the population between the classes, and especially the 'decline' in the proportion of Class V, has been believed to be larger than in fact it has been" [225]. There have actually been rather large shifts.

For example, between 1931 and 1991: RG Class 1 increased nearly four-fold, from 2 to 8% of the economically active male population, whilst RG Class V more than halved, falling from about 13 to about 5%. In the intermediate Classes II and IV from 1971 to 1981, the proportionate changes were +86 and −38% [217]. These are significant changes; the ratio of Class V to Class I has changed from 7.2 in 1931 to 3.6 in 1951 to 1.7 in 1971 and 1.4 in 1991. The shifts have been even larger in the 'at risk' age groups (Table 11.2).

Moreover, these movements had not previously been related to age. For example, between 1951 and 1981; Class 1 increased from 2.1 to 7.3% of the economically active males aged 25–34, (+248%), while Class V fell from 8.6 to 5.0% (−42%). Between 1951 and 1991 the relative size of

Table 11.2. *Percent distributions of economically active men by occupational class 1931–1991*

	I	*II*	*III*	*IV*	*V*	*All classes*
1931	1.8	12.0	47.8	25.5	12.9	100
1951	2.7	12.8	51.5	23.3	9.7	100
1971	5.0	18.2	50.5	18.0	8.4	100
1991	7.8	28.0	41.7	15.0	4.6	100

Source: Illsley [6] and own calculations from OPCS.

Occupational Class V to Class I aged 55–64 changed from 8.2 to 1.2%. Again, these are substantial changes over a 30-year period allowing for considerable changes in the composition of each class. Clearly, for classes defined in terms of an occupational classification (the classification used to demonstrate the 'unchanging' gap between the social classes), the balance is dynamic. Specifically, in the 'at-risk' age groups:

- The classes with high death rates now form a much smaller segment of our society.
- The classes with lower death rates form a much larger segment of society.
- The composition of each class, especially in terms of health status, might have changed substantially as a consequence, making it difficult to interpret a comparison of rates over time.

The impact these changes have on an assessment of inequalities in death depends upon the definition of inequality employed. A definition based solely in terms of class (assuming that class death rates do not change) leads to the conclusion that inequality is unchanged. It might also be argued that inequality has decreased, because a smaller proportion of the population is subject to the highest risks of death. In practice, class-specific death rates change for other reasons than their change in size.

A worked example

Table 11.3 compares changes in the infant mortality rates in Class 1 as compared to Class V. For both classes, rates fell sharply, but the fall was sharper in Class 1 until 1970–1972. Townsend and Davidson [213], interpreted the rates as diverging (the increasing 'gap'). Yet the *number* of infant deaths in Class 1 increased and the number in Class V was only 4% of its 1931 level.

In the last decade, the rates have fallen faster in Class V, but inequality, assessed in terms of the ratio of class death rates, is still large. If current

Table 11.3. *Infant mortality rates for Classes I and V*

Social Class	*1930–1932*	*1949–1953*	*1970–1972*	*1978–1979*	*1982*	*1996*
I	32	19	12	10	6.7	4.3
V	80	42	31	18	12.4	8.2

trends continue, the 'gap' is almost certain to widen, even though the number of deaths in Class V is shrinking because Class V is itself disappearing!

The message is two-fold:

- *There has been a very substantial change in class size.* Where it is possible to use a method that controls changes in class size (such as quintile method), this is preferable. Where this cannot be done, these changes should be taken into account routinely in any commentary upon the inequalities in health.[9]
- *These analyses have all been based on inequalities in death rates.* The usual ratio of rates can be derived from Table 11.3. The difference in ratios and the proportion of preventable deaths in Social Class V computed as the excess compared to Social Class I are shown in Part (a) of Table 11.4. All three have declined, but at different rates. Moreover, if inequalities in health were to be measured in terms of the numbers and proportion who survive rather than the numbers and rates of death, the picture is very different (Part (b) of Table 11.4).

The point is that as a negative outcome becomes more rare, it is more and more likely to occur disproportionately among the less advantaged groups. Conversely, as a valued outcome becomes relatively rarer, it is likely to be concentrated among the elite. This is a simple consequence of the statistical distributions [226], rather than another example of inequalities.

[9] The only thorough analysis is that of Pamuk [224] who also argues that inequalities in health (as measured by social class death rates before 65) have increased since the Second World War. She addresses the problems of changes in classification by experimenting with a uniform ranking across the 50 years, and the so-called 'numerator–denominator' problem by successively excluding the groups most likely to be affected. Her analysis shows whilst these two factors do make a difference, they cannot account for the trends. However, she is unable to take account of occupational selection accompanying changes in class size using this method and the same is true for the frequently quoted analysis of Koskinen [227]. More importantly, in this context, her analysis is once again restricted to social class death rates before 65 and therefore to only a small and decreasing fraction of all deaths.

Table 11.4. *Comparisons of trends in inequality between Social Classes I and V in terms of infant mortality and survival*

	1930–1932	*1978–1979*	*1984*
(a) Approach based on infant mortality rates (per 1000)			
Difference of rates (V − I)	44	8	6.5
Ratio of rates for V:I	2.5	1.8	2.0
Alternatively,			
Ratio of rates for I:V	0.43	0.56	0.5
And so,			
Proportion of preventable deaths in social class V	57%	44%	50%
(b) Approach based on rates of infant survival			
Survival of Social Class V (per 1000)	923	982	987
Survival of Social Class I (per 1000)	967	990	993.5
Ratio of survival rates V:I	0.95	0.99	0.993
Percentage possible improvement	5%	1%	0.7%

11.3.2 Social Selection

The process of social mobility discriminates in favour of the healthy and against the unhealthy [228]. This has been formalised in terms of a theoretical model, showing how under various assumptions, social class differences in health could occur simply as a result of the healthy moving up and the unhealthy moving down the social scale [229].

Any selection effect, whether directly because of health or indirectly because of factors associated with health, has been claimed to be *marginal* because of two reasons. First, only a very small proportion of those seriously ill in adulthood had suffered downward mobility as a result of previous childhood illness. However, this is incorrect. Any of those who are downwardly mobile through illness in childhood are at risk of early death before 65, whilst those who are upwardly mobile have a smaller risk. The only obvious way of measuring risk is by health status. Given the relatively small numbers who die before 65 the issue is whether social mobility discriminates in favour of the healthy and against the unhealthy, by even a small amount. Data from the National Survey of Health and Development demonstrates both a shift in the balance of classes and how a gap of 3% in the incidence of serious illness has more than doubled to 7% by the process of selection [230]. Second, social mobility might discriminate indirectly between the healthy and the unhealthy according to characteristics associated with health, so that the interpretation in terms of social selection is flawed. This is a particularly complex issue. Sometimes, the 'selection' argument is produced without any justification.

Example

In discussions of the relative rates of self-reported illness according to occupation, order and sex from the GHS, it has been claimed that certain illness ratios may reflect selection factors as much as they do actual occupational hazards, and that the reason why men in clerical and related work have slightly raised ratios could suggest such selection factors, given that women in these occupations have low ratios. The consistently high ratios for both men and women in personal service and jobs involving repetitive assembling and packing are interpreted as reflecting the selection of people with chronic illness into occupations which are less physically demanding.

The first interpretation about the way in which poor people are selected into hazardous occupations is plausible and the inference about the selection of women into low-paid occupations is unexceptionable; but the authors do not support interpretation that the high ratios of long-standing illness in personal service reflect selection rather than the working conditions.

It is right to criticise any claim that all social class differences can be explained by selective mobility. But there is an effect which should not be ignored; the size of the effect could be substantial, but it cannot be estimated properly without a lifelong longitudinal study for one particular birth cohort.

11.3.3 Material and Structural Explanations

Material and structural explanations are amongst the most obvious, as those who live in bad housing, or with low incomes, have a lower quality of life in general and are therefore likely to have poorer health. The relationship is not as straightforward as this, however.

On a 'macro' level there is a seemingly clear statistical relationship between current resources and ill health or mortality: [231]

- Comparing several countries, a relationship has been demonstrated between mortality and GNP.
- There is a relationship between occupational grouping and age-adjusted death rates.

In addition, there is a temporal relationship between:

- Relative income and mortality on the basis of analyses of percentage changes in mean occupational earnings and occupation-specific death rates ($N = 22$).
- Between the level of state pensions and mortality among the elderly ($N = 16$).
- The narrowing of class differences in incomes and post-neonatal mortality.

Not only are these numbers very small, the correlations are at a very macro level and do not permit a causal inference. However, a connection between income and mortality does exist.

Which connection?

The problem is which connection? The relationship between health and poverty (or wealth) stretches over a long time span even considering only 'direct' effects. Health during early working years may well affect motivation and prospects for occupational and earnings mobility. And family background whilst a child, as well as own status in previous years, may well affect present health status.

In effect, there are three connections here, between:

- Current resources and health status.
- Socio-economic status in early adulthood and current health status.
- Childhood household resources and current health status.

The initial evidence on the long-term nature of these relationships came from the series of papers by Barker and Osmond [232–234]. They argued that "past differences in maternal health and physique and in the post-natal environment, particularly infant feeding, housing and overcrowding, may be determinants of current differences in adult mortality" [234].

The connection between unemployment and health

There has been extensive research about the disadvantages of being unemployed, much of which is 'ideological' in the sense that unemployment is assumed to be 'bad': (Box 28)

- Unemployment usually leads to a severe drop in income for those already in poorly paid jobs, usually with adverse consequences.
- However, the claim that unemployment per se has effects on physical health is rarely evidenced.
- Yet considerable effort is made to refute the existence of a 'healthy worker' effect, whereby ill health tends to be associated with job loss [235].
- Most studies show immediate short-term effects of unemployment on self-reported health which are diffused over time [236]; none of which have controlled for income [21].
- The most important and well-known evidence is the follow-up material from the OPCS longitudinal study, which show that unemployment is associated with a higher death rate in subsequent years.

Box 28

Employment kills?

Apart from the caveat that the observation of unemployment is based on one week in 1971 [19], the apparent *increase* in SMRs during the second five years after unemployment is curious. Perhaps, those unemployed in 1971 later took a badly paid job with poor working conditions – in other words, employment kills.

An opposite interpretation is supported by a longitudinal study from France, which compared mortality among men aged 55 to 65 between 1975 and 1980 [237]. The findings from this study suggest that:

- Mortality is higher for those not employed than for those in work.
- The difference is largest amongst those between 55 and 60 which, at the time, was below the usual age for retirement, except for civil servants.
- Among other occupational groups, the retired group had retired early, possibly for health reasons, and this is supported by the pattern of mortality according to previous occupation.

The British and French results appear, then, to have different interpretations which may of course be the result of 'selection effects', though such conclusions may be politically unacceptable. However, even the case for showing a direct connection between *unemployment* and (ill) health, is not robust.

Points to Remember

- Although ill health might *directly* play a part in job loss, unemployment can only indirectly affect health *through* poverty.
- Although the 'poverty' effect of being unemployed may be large, it is not limited to the status of unemployment.

Box 29

Does unemployment equal deprivation?

"It is, we believe, mistaken to treat being unemployed as part of the definition of deprivation. Even if many among this minority are deprived, some are not and the point is to find out how many are deprived rather than operate as if all were in that condition. It is the form their deprivation takes and not their status which has to be measured" [211].

11.3.4 Behavioural Explanations

The final group of explanations considered by the WGIH focussed on the behavioural patterns in different 'sub-cultures' in the U.K., with a particular focus upon the deleterious effects of alcohol and tobacco consumption. Regional concerns on diet and quality of food consumed were also raised.

Interpreting the Data Relating Alcohol and Tobacco Consumption with Death Rates

Materialist or structural explanations contend that the concentration of alcohol and tobacco consumption and households with inadequate diet is a consequence of poverty. The relation between alcohol and tobacco consumption and death rates over time is difficult to interpret because patterns of consumption have changed. Analysis of results from the GHS shows the variation in patterns of consumption over the 'lifetime' of the survey:

- The proportionate decline in cigarette smoking has been greater in non-manual than in manual workers.
- The SMRs from lung cancer have dropped by 20% for non-manual compared to 10% for manual workers.
- It is nevertheless still difficult to determine what the link is meant to be between smoking and deaths from lung cancer in the *same period.*

The Food Connection

Commenting on the report by Townsend et al. [211] on health inequalities in the Northern region, Edwina Currie, then junior Minister for Health, said:

> "I honestly don't think the problem has anything to do with poverty. My family grew up in Liverpool and they didn't have two beans, but as a result of good food, good family and good rest, they grew up fit and well. The problem very often is, I think, just ignorance . . ." (Hansard, 1986).

There is some evidence available about the ability of those who are relatively poor now to feed themselves as compared with previous periods.

Table 11.5 presents estimates of the cost of Seebohm Rowntree's Dietary and overall subsistence income. The following points should be noted:

- A scaling up of £31 (the cost of the 1950 basket today) gives an estimated subsistence income of £137.
- The relative proportion Rowntree allowed in 1950 for food (41%) was close to the weight given to food in the retail price index basket of goods used to calculate the RPI (35%).

Table 11.5. *The cost of the 1950 Dietary, its price index Rowntree's subsistence income level, the equivalent subsistence income, based on the relative weight assigned to food in the RPI, and the scales of social security benefit excluding rent*

Year	*Cost of 1950 dietary (£)*	*Index of cost of 1950 dietary (£)*	*Rowntree actual subsistence Income*[a] *(£)*	*Outdoor relief national assistance/SB/IS (£)*	*Equivalent subsistence incomelevel*[b] *(£)*
1899	0.97	100	1.08	–	–
1936	1.18	142	2.65	1.90	–
1950	2.17	244	5.76	4.43	6.20
1985	30.95	3191	–	90.00	106.75
1998	31.15	3216	–	139.00	137.00

[a] Rowntree included rent in his discussion of the poverty line in 1899 and 1936; in 1950, he estimated the subsistence income at £5.01 excluding rent, but we have added on the median rent of 15s paid by class 'A' and class 'B' families, which was also the average rent for five rooms plus a bathroom.
[b] 1950 estimates based on the weight of food in the average RPI (350/100); 1985 and 1998 estimates based on weight of food in expenditure patterns of lowest income quintiles in family expenditure surveys for those years (29 and 22.7%, respectively).

- The RPI averages across families of all incomes.
- The latest family expenditure survey shows that 5-person households in the lowest income bracket spend 29% of their budget on food (compared to 20% for all families).
- Applying this proportion to the £31 food cost gives an estimated subsistence income of £107.
- The level of supplementary benefit was about £90 for a family of five plus an average allowance for rent and rates of £24.60.

It may be clear from the above that despite several government claims to the contrary, it is actually difficult to buy the contemporary equivalent of Rowntree's 'no better than workhouse' diet, with important implications for the connection between poverty, poor diet, and ill health.

Our estimates

On this basis, the price of the 1950 Dietary, suggests that the same minimal basket of goods would cost £31.15 today. In the previous exercise in 1985, the estimated cost was £30.95 – only 20 pence less. We attribute the small difference from 1985 to the spread of relatively aggressive competition between supermarkets regardless of quality.

Rowntree's estimate of the minimum expenditure, including that on housing, necessary to enable a family with three children to subsist is given in column 4. The cost of the 1950 Dietary (£2.17) was only part of what Rowntree adjudged to be the poverty line. For the same family of two adults and three children, we have estimated an overall figure of £5.76 including rent. The column 5 gives the scale of social security benefit prevailing in the same years. Our estimates of what a family of five would require if they subsisted on Rowntree's 1950 Dietary is given in the last column. The present supplementary benefit levels allow about £139 for a family of five, (£79.00 + £17.30 + £17.30 + £25.35) plus a family premium of £11.05 rent and rates are paid in full up to a limit set locally (Table 11.5).

11.3.5 Income Inequality and Health Inequalities

The model for the association between income *inequality* and inequalities in health suggests that it is high levels of income inequalities throughout society – a polarisation of communities between concentrations of affluence and poverty – which lead in turn to social disorganisation and a deterioration of community involvement, values, and interpersonal trust within poorer, economically disadvantaged areas.

Wilkinson [18] argues that mortality in developed countries is affected more by relative than absolute living standards because:

- Mortality rates are related more closely to relative income within countries than to differences in absolute income between them.
- National mortality rates tend to be lowest in countries that have smaller income differences and thus have lower levels of *relative* deprivation.
- Most of the long-term rise in life expectancy seems unrelated to long-term economic growth rates.

Kawachi and Kennedy [238] suggest that the effect of greater income inequality may be mediated by:

- Under-investment in public or social goods such as public education and healthcare.
- Disruption of social cohesion and the erosion of social capital.
- Harmful psychological effect of social comparisons.

This process is argued to have serious deleterious psycho-social as well as material consequences, finding their broadest expression in the physical health of a community and its members, and its psychological health in terms of interpersonal and community relations – perhaps most graphically seen in high levels of crime such as vandalism, robberies and violent assaults.

Disparities are observed not only in higher total mortality rates as a whole, but also from specific pathologies such as coronary heart disease, malignant neoplasms, and homicide. Income inequality together with 'poverty' could therefore account for around 25% of state variations in overall mortality and over 50% of the variation in homicide rates [238].

The Wilkinson thesis has become rather a proxy for the 'psycho-social' explanation as a whole, as it uses predominantly psycho-social pathways for the explanation of how the dynamics of local community interactions influence social cohesion and thereby health. There is a rather inevitable gradient between the level of the community as a whole and of the individual who lives in it. A number of different studies have explored aspects of this spectrum of psycho-social influence, some dealing more explicitly with psycho-social mechanisms as they influence individuals [239,240].

Although it is near impossible to divorce individual psycho-social explanations for ill health from social capital explanations, as it is to divorce the individuals themselves from the communities in which they live, the psycho-social explanations for the persistence of health inequalities is gaining much currency in recent years. The pathways that mediate these relationships, however, prove more difficult to determine precisely. Whilst wide inequalities in income (or wealth) mean that there are more (relatively) poor people who are also ill, it is (relative) poverty not the inequalities in income that is the cause.

11.3.6 Inequalities in Avoidable Death

There have been attempts to associate relative distribution of healthcare resources with early death and social deprivation, like unemployment with mortality. This has been proposed as an explanation for inequalities in health rather than inequalities in access to healthcare.

It is almost impossible to specify a complete model linking together all the factors that play a part in the process. The problem is illustrated in Figure 11.1. We need to be able to estimate the weight that should be attached to each arrow, but without a precise specification of the causal links being proposed and of the lag structure (the delay between a cause and its effect). It is impossible to make any more definitive statements than that we know certain conditions are associated with early death (Table 11.6).

11.4 Summary and Conclusions

Although many categories have been used to sub-divide populations when investigating health inequalities, social class has perhaps received

Figure 11.1. *Factors associated with mortality that might be considered in health service resource allocation.*

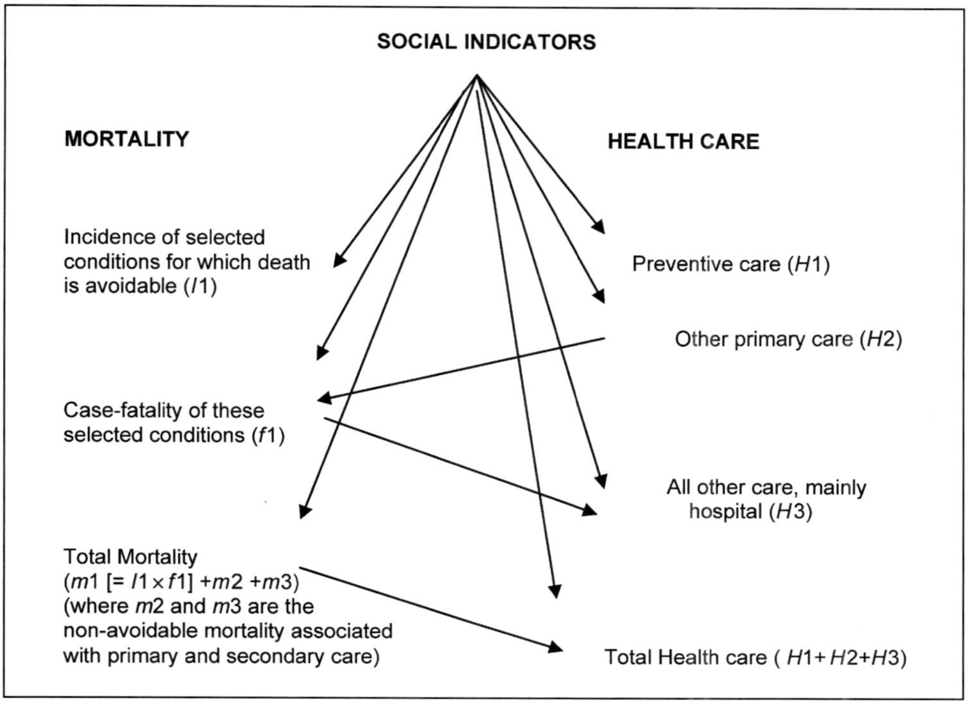

the most attention in the U.K. This may simply be because it has provided the longest lasting set of data on social differentiation. Many mechanisms have been advanced to account for variations in health, and mortality, with class. Most of these can be understand within the

Table 11.6. *Mechanisms investigated for explaining differences in health between classes*

Mechanism	*References*
Environment exposures	[241–247]
Occupational exposures	[248,249]
Personal risk factors, e.g. smoking, alcohol	[250–256]
Genetic difference	[257]
Social stress/Biological fight-or-flight response	[66,258,259]
Differences in disease detection/differences in survival	[260–262]
Disease related social mobility/health-related selection in employment	[263–265,76,266–268]
Nutrition	[269,270]
Early life conditions	[271,272]
Community structure	[273–277]
Race and/or gender	[278–282]

framework described in this chapter and the four approaches identified by the Black Report:

- Artefactuality (socio-economic class and SMRs).
- Social selection.
- Material and structural.
- Health-related behavioural.

We have also described a more recent psycho-social perspective (Section 11.3.5). And we have introduced a model that might be used to associate the distribution of healthcare resources with inequalities in health (Section 11.3.6).

These perspectives, and the differences between them, are fundamental to understanding reported inequalities in health. Many of the health and social surveys, health questionnaires, and indexes described in this book have been developed in the context these approaches. Again, it is hard to understate the importance of analytically separating methods and results, in order to assess the influence of the former on the latter.

References

[1] Szreter SRS. The genesis of the Registrar General's social classification of occupations. *Br J Sociol* 1984;*35*:522–46.

[2] Black. DHSS, Inequalities in Health, report of a research working group, London: DHSS, 1980.

[3] Atkinson AB. *Measuring inequality and differing social judgements*. London: London School of Economics; 1989.

[4] Bowling A. *Measuring health: a review of quality of life measurement scales*, 2nd ed. Buckingham: Open University Press; 1997.

[5] Wilkin D, Hallam L and Doggett M-A. *Measures of need and outcome for primary care*. Oxford: Oxford University Press; 1992.

[6] Morris R and Carstairs V. Which deprivation? a comparison of selected deprivation indexes. *J Public Health Med* 1991;*13*(4):318–26.

[7] Kunst AE and Mackenbach JP. *Measuring socio-economic inequalities in health*. Geneva: WHO; 1995.

[8] Valkonen T, et al. *Socioeconomic mortality differences in Finland 1981–90*. Helsinki: Statistics Finland; 1993.

[9] Wagstaff A, Paci P and Doorslaer E. On the measurement of inequalities in health. *Social Sci Med* 1991;*33*:545–57.

[10] Blaxter M. Self-definition of health status and consulting rates in primary care. *Quarterly J Social Affairs* 1985;*I*(2):131–71.

[11] MacIntyre S. The patterning of health by social position in contemporary Britain: directions for sociological research. *Social Sci Med* 1986;*23*(4):393–415.

[12] Hechter M. *Internal colonialism: the Celtic fringe in British national development*. NJ Transaction: New Brunswick; 1975 (1999 originally published in 1975).

[13] Harrison L, Carr-Hill R and Sutton M. Consumption and harm: drinking patterns of the Irish, the English and the Irish in England. *Alcohol Alcoholism* 1993;*28*(6):715–23.

[14] Balarajan R, Balsa L. Mortality amongst immigrants in England and Wales 1979–83. In: Britten M, editor. *Mortality and geography. A review in the mid nineteen eighties*. OPCS Series, DS8, No. 9, London: HMSO; 1990.

[15] Britten M. *Mortality and geography: a review in the mid ninety eighties*. OPCS Series, DS8, No.9, London: HMSO; 1990.

[16] Raleigh VS and Balarajan R. Suicide and self-burning among Indians and West-Indians in England and Wales. *Br J Psychiatry* 1992;*161*:365–8.

[17] Bartley M, Blane D and Davey Smith G. Introduction. Beyond the Black Report. In: Bartley M, Blane D, Davey Smith G, editors. *The sociology of health inequalities*. Oxford: Blackwell; 1998. p. 1–16.

[18] Wilkinson RG. *Unhealthy Societies: The afflictions of inequality*. London: Routledge; 1996.

[19] Fox AJ and Goldblatt PO. *Socio-demographic mortality differentials: longitudinal study 1971–75*. OPCS, Series LS No. 1, London: HMSO; 1982.

[20] Kitagawa EM and Hauser PM. *Differential mortality in the US: a study in socioeconomic epidemiology*. Cambridge, MA: Harvard University Press; 1973.

[21] Carr-Hill RA. Whither (research on) unemployment. In: Roberts B, Gallie D, Finnegan R, editors. *New approaches to economic life*. Manchester: Manchester University Press; 1985.

[22] Hussmanns R, Mehran F and Verma V. *Surveys of economically active population, employment, unemployment and underemployment – an ILO manual on concepts and methods*. Geneva: International Labour Office; 1990.

[23] Sorrentino C. International comparisons of unemployment indicators. *Monthly Labour Rev* 1993;*116*:3–24.

[24] Stevenson THC. The vital statistics of wealth and poverty. *J R Stat Soc* 1928;*XCI*:207–30.

[25] Dale A and March C. *The 1991 census user's guide*. London: HMSO; 1993.

[26] Marang-van de Mheen PJ, Davey Smith G, Hart CL and Gunning-Schepers LJ. Socioeconomic differentials in mortality among men within Great Britain: time trends and contributory causes. *J Epidemiol Community Health* 1998;*52*(4):214–8.

[27] Davey Smith G, Hart C, Hole D, MacKinnon P, Gillis C, Watt G, Blane D and Hawthorne V. Education and occupational social class: which is the more important indicator of morality risk? *J Epidemiol Community Health* 1998;*52*(3):153–60.

[28] Barnett E, Armstrong DL and Casper ML. Social class and premature mortality among men: a method for state-based surveillance. *Am J Public Health* 1997;*87*(9):1521–5.

[29] Gregorio DI, Walsh SJ and Paturzo D. The effects of occupation-based social position on mortality in a large American cohort. *Am J Public Health* 1997;*87*(9):1472–5.

[30] Drever F, Whitehead M and Roden M. Current patterns and trends in male mortality by social class (based on occupation). *Population Trends* 1996;*Winter*(86):15–20.

[31] Harding S. Social class differences in mortality of men: recent evidence from the OPCS longitudinal study. Office of Population Censuses and Surveys. *Population Trends* 1995;*Summer*(80):31–7.

[32] Minder CE and Beer-Porizek V. Cancer mortality of Swiss men by occupation, 1979–1982. *Scand J Work Environ Health* 1992;*18*(Suppl 3):1–27.

[33] Marmot MG, Davey Smith G, Stanfield S, Patel C, North F, Head J, White L, Brunner E, Feeney A. Health inequalities among British civil servants: The Whitehall II study. *Lancet* 1991;*337*:1387–93.

[34] Hadden WC. Annotation: the use of educational attainment as an indicator of socioeconomic position. *Am J Public Health* 1996;*86*(11):1525–6.

[35] Sorlie PD, Backlund E and Keller JB. US mortality by economic, demographic, and social characteristics: the national longitudinal mortality study. *Am J Public Health* 1995;*85*(7):949–56.

[36] Leclerc A, Pietri F, Boitel L, Chastang JF, Carval P, Blondet M. Level of education, lifestyle, and morbidity in two groups of white collar workers. *J Epidemiol Community Health* 1992;*46*(4):403–8.

[37] Winkleby MA, Fortmann SP and Barrat DC. Social class disparities in risk factors for disease – 8 year prevalence patterns by level of education. *Prevent Med* 1990;*19*(1):1–12.

[38] Kaufman JS, Long AE, Liao Y, Cooper RS and McGee DL. The relation between income and mortality in US blacks and whites. *Epidemiology* 1998;*9*(2):147–55.

[39] Lundberg O and Fritzell J. Income distribution, income change and health: on the importance of absolute and relative income for health status in Sweden. *WHO Regional Publications. European Series* 1994;*54*:37–58, discussion 123–128.

[40] Wannamethee SG and Shaper AG. Socioeconomic status within social class and mortality: a prospective study in middle-aged British men. *Int J Epidemiol* 1997;*26*:532–41.

[41] Massey DS. The age of extremes: concentrated affluence and poverty in the twenty-first century. *Demography* 1996;*33*(4):395–412, discussion, 413–416.

[42] Hart N. Inequalities in health: the individual versus the environment. *J R Stat Soc* 1986;*149*(3):228–46, Series A (General).

[43] Helmert U and Shea S. Social inequalities and health status in Western Germany. *Public Health* 1994;*108*(5):341–56.

[44] Faggiano F, Zanetti R and Costa G. Cancer risk and social inequalities in Italy. *J Epidemiol Community Health* 1994;*48*(5):447–52.

[45] Hart CL, Smith GD and Blane D. Social mobility and 21 year mortality in a cohort of Scottish men. *Social Sci Med* 1998;*47*(8):1121–30.

[46] Power C and Mathews S. Origins of health inequalities in a national population sample. *Lancet* 1997;*350*:1584–9.

[47] West P. Unhealthy societies: the afflictions of inequality. Comment on Wilkinson 1996. *Sociol Health* 1997;*19*(5):668–70.

[48] Smith GD, Hart C, Blane D, Gillis C and Hawthorne V. Lifetime socioeconomic position and mortality: prospective observational study. *Br Med J* 1997;*314*:547–52.

[49] Wannamethee SG, Whincup PH, Shaper G and Walker M. Influence of fathers' social class on cardiovascular disease in middle-aged men. *Lancet* 1996;*348*(9037): 1259–63.

[50] Wilkinson RG. Commentary: Income inequality summarises the health burden of individual relative deprivation. *Br Med J* 1997;*314*:1724–7.

[51] Judge K. Income distribution and life expectancy: a critical appraisal. *Br Med J* 1995;*311*:1282–5.

[52] Robert SA. Community-level socioeconomic status effects on adult health. *J Health Soc Behav* 1998;*39*(1):18–37.

[53] Hayward MD, Pienta AM and McLaughlin DK. Inequality in men's mortality: the socioeconomic status gradient and geographic context. *J Health Soc Behav* 1997;*38*(4):313–30.

[54] Diez-Roux AV, Nieto FJ, Muntaner C, Tyroler HA, Comstock GW, Shahar E, Cooper LS, Watson RL and Szklo M. Neighborhood environments and coronary heart disease: a multilevel analysis. *Am J Epidemiol* 1997;*146*(1):48–63.

[55] Woodward M. Small area statistics as markers for personal social status in the Scottish heart health studies. *J Epidemiol Community Health* 1996;*50*(5):570–6.

[56] Kaplan GA. People and places: contrasting perspectives on the association between social class and health. *Int J Health Services* 1996;*26*(3):507–19.

[57] Hyndman JC, Holman CD, Hockey RL, Donovan RJ, Corti B, Rivera J. Misclassification of social disadvantage based on geographical areas: comparison of postcode and collector's district analyses. *Int J Epidemiol* 1995;*24*(1):165–76.

[58] Starrin B, Hagquist C, Larsson G and Svensson PG. Community types, socio-economic structure and IHD mortality – a contextual analysis based on Swedish aggregate data. *Social Sci Med* 1993;*36*(12):1569–78.

[59] Humphreys K, Carr-Hill R. Area variations in health outcomes: artefact or ecology. *Int J Epidemiol* 1991;*20*(1):251–8.

[60] Krieger N. Women and social class: a methodological study comparing individual, household, and census measures as predictors of black/white differences in reproductive history. *J Epidemiol Community Health* 1991;*45*(1):35–42.

[61] Logue EE and Jarjoura D. Modeling heart disease mortality with census tract rates and social class mixtures. *Social Sci Med* 1990;*31*:545–50.

[62] Kawachi I and Kennedy BP. Socioeconomic determinants of health: Health and social cohesion: why care about income inequality? *Br Med J* 1997;*314*(7086):1037–41.

[63] Ostergren PO, Lindbladh E, Isacsson SO, Odeberg H and Svensson SE. Social network, social support and the concept of control – a qualitative study concerning the validity of certain stressor measures used in quantitative social epidemiology. *Scand J Social Med* 1995;*23*(2):95–102.

[64] Arber S. Class, paid employment and family roles: making sense of structural disadvantage, gender and health status. *Social Sci Med* 1991;*32*(4):425–36.

[65] Marmot MG, Bosma H, Hemingway H, Brunner E and Stansfeld S. Contribution of job control and other risk factors to social variations in coronary heart disaease incidence. *Lancet* 1997;*350*:235–9.

[66] Wickrama KA, Lorenz FO, Conger RD, Matthews L and Elder Jr GH. Linking occupational conditions to physical health through marital, social, and intrapersonal processes. *J Health Soc Behav* 1997;*38*(4):363–75.

[67] Smith GD and Harding S. Is control at work the key to socioeconomic gradients in mortality? *Lancet* 1997;*350*(9088):1369–70, [Letter].

[68] Benzeval M, Judge K and Smaje C. Beyond class, race and ethnicity: deprivation and health in Britain. *Health Services Res* 1995;*30*(1 Pt 2):163–77.

[69] Thomas VG. Using feminist and social structural analysis to focus on the health of poor women. *Women Health* 1994;*22*(1):1–15.

[70] McCarron PG, Smith GD and Womersley JJ. Deprivation and mortality in Glasgow: changes from 1980 to 1992. *Br Med J* 1994;*309*(6967):1481–2.

[71] Sloggett A and Joshi H. Higher mortality in deprived areas – community or personal disadvantage. *Br Med J* 1994;*309*:1470–4.

[72] Black D. Deprivation and health. *Br Med J* 1993;*307*(6919):1630–1.

[73] Charlton BG. Social deprivation and health. Wealth redistribution has its price. *Br Med J* 1993;*307*(6917):1499.

[74] Carstairs V and Morris R. Deprivation and health in Scotland. *Health Bull* 1990; *48*(4):162–75.

[75] Novak T. The class analysis of poverty: a response to Erik Olin Wright. *Int J Health Services* 1996;*26*(1):187–95.

[76] Bartley M and Owen C. Relation between socioeconomic status, employment and health during economic change, 1973–93. *Br Med J* 1996;*313*:445–9.

[77] Masterson-Allen S and Brown P. Public reaction to toxic waste contamination: analysis of a social movement. *Int J Health Services* 1990;*20*(3):485–500.

[78] Kerr NL. Applied perspectives on social and temporal dilemmas – an introduction. *Social Behav* 1990;*5*(4):201–5.

[79] Hoggart R, A local habitation. Life and times, vol. 1. London: Chatto and Windus; 1988, pp. 1918–1940.

[80] Cochrane R. *The social creation of mental illness*. London: Longman; 1983.

[81] Fanning DM. Families in flats. *Br Med J* 1967;*4*(516):382–6.

[82] Jephcott P. *Homes in high flats*. Edinburgh: Oliver and Boyd; 1971.

[83] Kasl SV. Strategies of research on economic instability and health. *Psychol Med* 1982;*12*:637–49.

[84] Marsh A. *Home sweet home?: the impact of poor housing on health*. Bristol: Policy Press; 1999.

[85] Smith SJ and Mallinson S. The problem with social housing: discretion, accountability and the welfare ideal. *Policy Politics* 1996;*24*(4):339–58.

[86] Montgomery SM, Bartley MJ, Cook DG and Wadsworth ME. Health and social precursors of unemployment in young men in Great Britain. *J Epidemiol Community Health* 1996;*50*(4):415–22.

[87] Strachan DP and Elton RA. Relationship between respiratory morbidity and the home environment. *Family Practitioner* 1986;*3*:137–42.

[88] Platt-Mills TAE and Chapman MD. Dust mites: immunology, allergic disease and environmental control. *J Allergy Clin Immunol* 1987;*80*(6):755–75.

[89] Burr ML, Mullins J, Merrett TG and Stott NC. Indoor moulds and asthma. *J Royal Soc Health* 1988;*108*(3):99–101.

[90] Platt SD, Martin CJ, Hunt SM and Lewis CW. Damp housing, mould growth and symptomatic health state. *Br Med J* 1989;*298*:1673–8.

[91] Hyndman SJ. Housing, dampness and health amongst British Bengalis in East London. *Social Sci Med* 1990;*30*(1):131–41.

[92] Dales RE, Burnett R and Zwanenburg H. Adverse health effects among adults exposed to home dampness and molds. *Am Rev Respir Disease* 1991;*143*(3):505–9.

[93] Sporik R and Platts-Mills TA. Epidemiology of dust-mite-related disease. *Exp Appl Acarology* 1992;*16*(1–2):141–51.

[94] Packer CJ, Fowle SE and Stuart-Brown S. Damp housing and adult health: results from a lifestyle study in Worcester, England. *J Epidemiol Community Health* 1994; *48*(6):555–9.

[95] Spengler J, Neas L, Nakai S, Dockery D, Speizer F, Ware J and Raizenne M. Respiratory symptoms and housing characteristics. *Int J Indoor Air Quality Climate* 1994;*4*(2):72–82.

[96] Verhoeff AP, van Strien RT, van Wijnen JH and Brunekreef B. Damp housing and childhood respiratory symptoms: the role of sensitization to dust mites and molds. *Am J Epidemiol* 1995;*141*(2):103–10.

[97] Hopton J and Hunt S. The health effects of improvement to housing: a longitudinal study. *Housing Studies* 1996;*11*(2):271–86.

[98] Williamson IJ, Martin CJ, McGill G, Monie RD and Fennerty AG. Damp housing and asthma: a case-control study. *Thorax* 1997;*52*(3):229–34.

[99] Weitzman M, Gortmaker S and Sobol A. Racial, social, and environmental risks for childhood asthma. *Am J Diseases Children* 1990;*144*(11):1189–94.

[100] Rona RJ and Chinn S. Lung function, respiratory illness, and passive smoking in British primary school children. *Thorax* 1993;*48*(1):21–5.

[101] Cook DG and Strachan DP. Health effects of passive smoking. 3. Parental smoking and prevalence of respiratory symptoms and asthma in school age children. *Thorax* 1997;*52*(12):1081–94.

[102] Ashmore JP, Krewski D, Zielinski JM, Jiang H, Semenciw R, Band PR. First analysis of mortality and occupational radiation exposure based on the national dose registry of Canada. *Am J Epidemiol* 1998;*148*(6):564–74.

[103] Collins KJ. Low indoor temperatures and mortality of the elderly. *Age Ageing* 1986;*15*(4):212–20.

[104] Blackman T, Melaugh M, Evason E and Woods R. Housing and health – a case study of two areas in West Belfast. *J Social Policy* 1989;*18*(1):1–26.

[105] Strachan DP and Sanders CH. Damp housing and childhood asthma – respiratory effects of indoor air temperature and relative humidity. *J Epidemiol Community Health* 1989;*43*:7–14.

[106] Collins KJ. Cold-and heat-related illnesses in the indoor environment. In: Burridge R, Ormandy D, editors. *Unhealthy housing: research, remedies and reform*. London: E and FN Spon; 1993.

[107] Shanks N and Smith SJ. Public policy and the health of homeless people. *Policy Politics* 1992;*20*(1):35–46.

[108] Bines W (1994) *The health of single homeless people* Centre for Housing Policy, University of York Discussion Paper no. 9.

[109] Conway J and Cole-Hamilton I. *Prescription for poor health: the crisis for homeless families*. London: London Food Commission; Maternity Alliance; SHAC; Shelter; 1988.

[110] Cloke P, Milbourne P, and Thomas C. (1994). *Lifestyles in rural England*. Rural Development Commission, Rural Research Report 18.

[111] McLaughlin BP. The rhetoric and the reality of rural disadvantage. *J Rural Studies* 1986;*2*:291–307.

[112] Mason S, Taylor R. *Tackling deprivation in rural areas: effective use of charity funding*. Cirencester: ACRE; 1990.

[113] Cloke PJ. An index of rurality of England and Wales. *Regional Studies* 1977;*II*:31–46.

[114] Office of population censuses and surveys, *Occupational mortality: decennial supplement 1979–80, 1982–83, Great Britain*. London: HMSO; 1986.

[115] Moscovice, IS. (1996). *Rural health networks: concepts, cases, and public policy*. Office of Rural Health Policy, University of Minnesota. Rockville, MD; Health Resources and Services Administration, U.S. Dept. of Health and Human Services.

[116] Lewis G, Booth M. Regional differences in mental health in Great Britain. *J Epidemiol Community Health* 1992;*46*(6):608–11.

[117] Durkheim E. *Suicide: a study in sociology*. London: Routledge Paul and Kegan; 1897.

[118] Bordieu P. The forms of capital. In: Richardson J G, editor. *Handbook of theory and research for the sociology of education*. New York: Greenwood; 1985. p. 241–358.

[119] Portes A. Social capital: its origins and applications in modern sociology. *Ann Rev Sociol* 1998;*24*:1–24.

[120] Putnam RD. *Making democracy work: Civic traditions in modern Italy*. Princeton, NJ: Princeton University Press; 1993.

[121] Putnam RD. Bowling alone: America's declining social capital. *Journal Democracy* 1995;*6*:65–78.

[122] Lowry P E. (1992). *Trade, development and social capability: an empirical analysis*. University of Maryland, PhD thesis.

[123] Bordieu P, Wacquant L. *Invitation to Reflexive Sociology*. Chicago: Chicago University Press; 1992.

[124] Sampson RJ, Raudenbush SW and Earls F. Neighbourhoods and violent crime: a multilevel study of collective efficacy. *Science* 1997;*277*:918–24.

[125] Runyan DK, Hunter WM, Socolar RR, Amaya-Jackson L, English D, Landsverk J and Dubowitz H, et al. Children who prosper in unfavourable environments: the relationship to social capital. *Paediatrics* 1998;*101*(1):12–18.

[126] Hunter A. The loss of community: an empirical test through replication. *Am Sociological Rev* 1975;*40*:537–52.

[127] Riger S and Lavrakas PJ. Community ties: patterns of attachment and social interaction in urban neighbourhoods. *Am J Community Psychology* 1981;*9*:55–66.

[128] Unger D and Wandersmann A. Neighboring and its role in block organization: an exploratory report. *Am J Community Psychology* 1983;*11*:291–300.

[129] Buckner JC. The development of an instrument to measure neighbourhood cohesion. *Am J Community Psychology* 1988;*16*:771–91.

[130] Perkins DD, Florin P, Rich RC, et al. Participation and the social and physical environment of neighbourhood blocks: crime and community context. *Am J Community Psychology* 1990;*18*:83–115.

[131] Unger D and Wundersmann A. The importance of neighbours: the social cognitive and affective components of neighbouring. *Am J Community Psychology* 1985; *13*:139–69.

[132] Lochner K, Kawachi I and Kennedy BP. Social capital: a guide to its measurement. *Health Place* 1999;*5*:259–70.

[133] Whitley E, Gunnell DJ, Dorling S and Davey Smith G. Ecological study of social fragmentation, pverty and suicide. *BMJ* 1999; *319*:1034–1037.

[134] Campbell C, Wood R and Kelly M (1999). Social capital and Health Education Authority. http://www.had-online.org.uk/downloads/pdfs/socialcapital health.pdf.

[135] Boreham C, Twisk J, Neville C, Savage M, Murray L and Gallagher A. Associations between physical fitness and activity patterns during adolescence and cardiovascular risk factors in young adulthood: the Northern Ireland Young Hearts Project. *Int J Sports Med* 2002;*23*(Suppl 1):S22–6.

[136] Cox BD, Blaxter M and Buckle ALJ, et al. *The health and lifestyle survey*. London: Health Promotion Research Trust; 1987.

[137] Gaffey WR. A critique of the standardised mortality ratio. *J Occup Med* 1976;*18*:157–60.

[138] Inskip H, Beral V and Fraser P, et al. Methods for age-adjustment of rates. *Stat Med* 1983;*2*:455–66.

[139] Prior L. Making sense of mortality. *Sociol Health Illness* 1985;*7*(2):220–35.

[140] Online: www.data-archive.ac.uk The labour force survey, data archive, University of Essex.

[141] Wade DT. *Measurement in neurological rehabilitation*. Oxford: Oxford University Press; 1992.

[142] McDowell I and Newell C. *Measuring health: a guide to rating scales and questionnaires*. Oxford: Oxford University Press; 1996, (and earlier editions).

[143] Bowling A. *Measuring disease: a review of disease-specific quality of life measurement scales*, 2nd ed. Buckingham: Open University Press; 2001.

[144] Mahoney FL and Barthel DW. Functional evaluation; the Barthel index. *Maryland State Med* 1965;*14*:61–5.

[145] Jette AM and Denisten OL. Inter-observer reliability of a functional status assessment instrument. *J Chronic Dis* 1978;*31*:573–80.

[146] Bergner M, Bobbitt RA, Kressel A, Pollard WE, Gilson BS and Morris JR. The Sickness Impact Profile: conceptual formulation and methodology for the development of a health status measure. *Int J Health Services* 1976;*6*:393–415.

[147] Patrick DL and Peach H. *Disablement in the community*. Oxford: Oxford University Press; 1989.

[148] Peach H, Green S, Locker D, Darby S and Patrick DL. Evaluation of a postal screening questionnaire to identify the physically disabled. *Int Rehabil Med* 1980;*2*:189–93.

[149] Fries JF, Spitz PW, Kraines RG and Holman HR. Measurement of patient outcome in arthritis. *Arthritis Rheumatism* 1980;*17*:137–45.

[150] Leavitt F, Garron DC. Validity of a back pain classification scale for detecting psychological disturbanceas measured by the MMPI. *J Clin Psychology* 1980;*36*:186–9.

[151] Meenan RF and Mason JH. *AIMS2 users' guide*. Boston, MA: Boston University School of Medicine, Department of Public Health; 1990.

[152] Zung WWK. The self-rating pain and distress scale. *Psychosomatics* 1983;*24*:887–94.

[153] Kahn RL, Goldfarb AI and Pollack M, et al. Brief objective measures for the determination of mental status in the aged. *Am J Psychiatry* 1960;*117*:326–8.

[154] Gurland B, Kuriansky J, Sharpe L, Simon R, Stiller P and Birkett P. The comprehensive assessment and referral evaluation (CARE)-rationale, development and reliability. *Int J Ageing Human Dev* 1977;*8*(1):9–42.

[155] Copeland JRM, Kelleher MH and Kellet JM, et al. A semi-structured clinical interview for the assessment of diagnosis and mental state in the elderly: the geriatric mental state test. Schedule 1: development and reliability. *Psychol Med* 1976;*16*:89–99.

[156] Pfeiffer. A short psychiatric evaluation schedule: A new 15 item monotonic scale indicative of functional psychiatric disorder (abstract). *The Gerontologist* 1975;*15*:34.

[157] Pfeiffer E, editor. *Multidimensional functional assessment: the OARS methodology. A manual*. Durham, N. Carolina: Duke University, Center for the Study of Aging and Human Development; 1975.

[158] Ebmeier KP, Beson JAO and Eagles JN, et al. Continuing care of the demented elderly in Inverurie. *Health Bull* 1988;*46*:32–41.

[159] Wilson LA and Brass W. Cognitive Functioning: Brief assessment of the mental state in geriatric domiciliary practice: the usefulness of the mental status questionnaire. *Age Ageing* 1973;*2*:92–101.

[160] Hodgkinson HM. Evaluation of a mental test score for assessment of mental impairment in the elderly. *Age Ageing* 1972;*1*:233–8.

[161] Carroll BJ and Feinberg M and Smouse PE, et al. The Carroll rating scale for depression. I. Development, reliability and validation. *Br J Psychiatry* 1981;*138*:194–200.

[162] Hamilton M. Development of a rating scale for primary depressive illness. *Br J Soc Clin Psychiatry* 1967;*6*:278–96.

[163] Goldberg DP. *General health questionnaire – current diagnosable psychiatric disorders*. London: Oxford University Press; 1972.

[164] Beck AT, Ward CH, Mendelson M, Mock J and Erbaugh J. An instrument for measuring depression. *Arch Gen Psychiatry* 1961;*4*:61–571.

[165] Zung WWK. A self rating depression scale. *Arch Gen Psychiatry* 1965;*12*:63–70.
[166] Ware JE, Johnson SA, Davies-Avery A and Brook RH. *Conceptualisation and measurement of health for adults in the health insurance study*. Mental health, vol. 3. Santa Monica, CA: Rand Corporation; 1979.
[167] Katz MM and Lyerly SS. Methods for measuring adjustment and social behaviour in the community: 1. Rationale, description, discriminative validity and scale development. *Psychological Reports* 1963;*13*:503–35, Monograph, (Suppl.).
[168] Feeny D, Barr RD and Furlong W, et al. Quality of life of the treatment process in paediatric oncology: an approach to measurment. In: Osoba D, editor. *Effect of cancer on quality of life*. Boston, MA: CRC Press; 1991.
[169] Rakos RF, Grodek MV and Mack KK. The impact of a self-administered behavioral intervention program on pediatric asthma. *J Psychosomatic Res* 1985;*29*(1):101–8.
[170] Usherwood TP, Scrimgeour A and Barber JH. Questionnaire to measure perceived symptoms and disability in asthma. *Arch Disease Childhood* 1990;*65*(7):779–81.
[171] Medical outcomes trust. (1993). Medical outcomes trust instruments. Medical outcomes trust bulletin, 1:1. MOT: Boston, MA
[172] Aaronson NK. The EORTC QLC-C30: a quality of life instrument for use in international clinical trials in oncology (abstract). *Qual Life Res* 1993;*2*:51.
[173] Aaronson NK, Bullinger M and Ahmedzai S. A modular approach to quality of life assessment in cancer clinical trials. *Recent Results Cancer Res* 1988;*111*:231–49.
[174] Sprangers MAG, Cull A and Bjordal K, et al. The European organisation for research and treatment of cancer approach to quality of life assessment: guidelines for developing questionnaire modules. *Qual Life Res* 1993;*2*:287–95.
[175] de Haes JCGM, van Ostrom MA and Welvaart K. The effect of radical and conserving surgery on the quality of life of early breast cancer patients. *Eur J Surg Oncol* 1986;*12*:337–42.
[176] Fayers PM and Jones DR. Measuring and analysing quality of life in cancer clinical trials: a review. *Stat Med* 1983;*2*:429–46.
[177] Schipper H, Clinch J, McMurray A and Levitt M. Measuring the quality of life of cancer patients: The functional living index – cancer: Development and validation. *J Clin Oncol* 1984;*2*:472–83.
[178] Ganz PA, Schag CAC and Kahn B, et al. The CARES: a generic measure of health related quality of life for patients with cancer. *Qual Life Res* 1992;*1*:19–29.
[179] Selby P. Measurment of the quality of life: The particular problems of patients with cancer. In: Hopkins A, editor. *Measures of the quality of life*. London: Royal College of Physicians; 1992.
[180] Padilla GV, Mishel MH and Grant MM. Uncertainty, appraisal and quality of life. *Qual Life Res* 1992a;*1*:155–65.
[181] Padilla GV, Grant MM and Ferrell B. Nursing research into quality of life. *Qual Life Res* 1992b;*1*:341–8.
[182] Hyland ME, Finnis S and Irvine SH. A scale for assessing quality of life in adult asthma sufferers. *J Psychosomatic Res* 1991;*35*:99–110.
[183] Marks GB, Dunn SM and Woolcock AJ. A scale for the measurement of quality of life in adults with asthma. *J Clin Epidemiol* 1992;*45*:461–72.
[184] Bone M, et al. *Health expectancy and its uses*. London: HMSO; 1995.
[185] Williams A. Science or marketing? A commentary on 'World Health at 2000'. *Health Economics* 2001;*10*:93–100.
[186] Kind P and Rosser R. A scale of valuations of states of illness; is there a social consensus? *Int J Epidemiol* 1978;*7*(4):347–58.
[187] Carr-Hill RA. Health related quality of life measurement – Euro style. *Health Policy* 1992;*20*(3):321–8, discussion 329–332.
[188] Blaxter M. *Health and lifestyle*. London: Tavistock/Routledge; 1990.

[189] Wright (1986). *Age, sex an health: a summary of findings from the York Health Evaluation Survey*. University of York, Centre for Health Economics, Discussion Paper 15.
[190] Gordon D and Forrest R. *People and places 2: social and economic distinctions in England*. Bristol: SAUS; 1995.
[191] Mack J and Lansley S. *Poor Britain*. London: George Allen and Unwin; 1985.
[192] Carr-Hill R. (1994). *Measuring resource inadequacy*. In mission report for World Bank, Ivory Coast, (mimeo).
[193] Lee P, Murie A and Gordon D. *Area measures of deprivation: a study of current methods and best practices in the identification of poor areas in Great Britain*. Birmingham: University of Birmingham; 1995.
[194] Nunnally. *Psychometric theory*, 2nd ed. New York: McGraw Hill; 1978.
[195] Streiner DL and Norman GR. *Health measurement scales – a practical guide to their development and use*. Oxford: Oxford University Press; 1995.
[196] Nunnally. *Introduction to psychological measurement (a major revision of tests and measurements)*. New York: McGraw Hill; 1970.
[197] O'Reilly, D. (2000). Standard indicators of deprivation: do they disadvantage older people? Unpublished ms.
[198] Jones IL and Cameron D. Social class analysis – an embarrassment to epidemiology. *Community Med* 1984;*6*:37–46.
[199] Gordon D. Census based deprivation indexes: their weighting and validation. *J Epidemiol Community Health* 1995;*49*(Suppl. 2):S39–S44.
[200] Kearns A, Gibb K and Mackay D. Area deprivation in Scotland: a new assessment. *Urban Studies* 2000;*37*(9):1535–60.
[201] Townsend. Deprivation. *J Social Policy* 1987;*16*:124–46.
[202] Townsend P, Philimore P and Beattie A. *Health and deprivation: inequality and the North*. London: Croom Helm; 1988.
[203] Carstairs V and Morris R. Deprivation and Mortality: an alternative to social class? *Community Med* 1989a;*11*(3):210–9.
[204] Carstairs V and Morris R. Deprivation: explaining difference in mortality between Scotland and England and Wales. *Br Med J* 1989b;*299*:886–9.
[205] Carstairs V and Morris R. *Deprivation and health in Scotland*. Aberdeen: Aberdeen University Press; 1991.
[206] Saunders J. Weighted census-based deprivation indexes: their use in small areas. *J Public Health Med* 1998;*20*(3):253–60.
[207] Aveyard P, Manaseki S and Chambers J. The relationship between mean birth weight and poverty using the Townsend deprivation score and the Super Profile classification system. *Public Health* 2002;*116*(6):308–14.
[208] Hays RD and Hadorn D. Responsiveness to change: an aspect of validity. *Qual Life Res* 1992;*1*(1):73–5.
[209] Jenkinson C. Quality of life measurement: does it have a place in routine clinical assessment? *J Psychosomatic Res* 1994;*38*(5):377–81.
[210] Goldthorpe J. Women and class analysis: a reply to the replies. *Sociology* 1984;*18*:491–9.
[211] Townsend P, Phillimore P and Beattie A. *Inequalities in health in the northern region*. Report to Nth RHA, Bristol: Bristol University; 1986.
[212] SeptEtzioni A and Lehman EW. Some dangers in 'valid' social measurement. *Ann Am Acad Political Social Sci* 1967;*1967*:1–15.
[213] Townsend P and Davidson N. *Inequalities in health: the Black Report*. London: Penguin; 1982.
[214] Bebbington A (1996) *Synthetic estimation methods for resource allocation formulae*. University of Kent at Canterbury. Personal Social Services Research Unit: Discussion Paper1203/3

[215] Turvey K. (1995). *Needs based planning. Use of information from individual assessments to develop population estimates of need and use of resources*. University of Kent at Canterbury. Personal Social Services Research Unit: Discussion Paper no 1136.

[216] Dixon P and Carr-Hill R. *The NHS and its customers II. Customer feedback surveys – an introduction to survey methods. Centre for health economics*. York: Centre for Health Economics; 1989.

[217] Illsley R. Occupational class, selection and the production of inequalities in health. *Quarterly J Social Affairs* 1986;*2*(2):151–65.

[218] Carr-Hill R. The measurement of inequities in health: lessons from the British experience. *Social Sci Med* 1990;*31*:393–404.

[219] Le Grand J. *Inequalities in health: the human capital approach*. Welfare state programme pamphlet no. 1, London: London School of Economics; 1985.

[220] Brown MC. Using Gini-style indexes to evaluate the spatial patterns of health practitioners: theoretical considerations and an application based on Alberta data. *Social Sci Med* 1994;*38*(9):1243–56.

[221] Wilkinson RG. Commentary: Income inequality summarises the health burden of individual relative deprivation. *Br Med J* 1997;*314*:1724–7.

[222] Murray GD. Promoting good research practice. *Statistical Methods Med Res* 2000;*9*(1):17–24.

[223] Preston SH, et al. Effect of industrialisation and urbanisation on mortality in developed countries. *Solicited Papers 2*. IUSSP 19th International Population Conference; 1981.

[224] Pamuk ER. Social class and inequality in mortality from 1921 to 1972 in England and Wales. *Population Studies* 1985;*39*:17–31.

[225] Department of Health and Social Security (DHSS), *Inequalities in health. The Black Report*. London: HMSO; 1980.

[226] Scanlan, J. (2002). The misunderstood relationship between declining mortality and increasing racial and social disparities in mortality rates. Presented at “Making a Difference: Is the Health Gap Widening?” Oslo Conference, Oslo, Norway, May14, 2001.

[227] Koskinen S. *Time trends in cause-specific mortality by occupational class in England and Wales*. Proceedings of IUSSP Conference at Florence, Florence: IUSSP; June 1988, pp. 1–41.

[228] Illsley R. Social class and selection and class differences in relation to stillbirths and infant deaths. *Br Med J* 1955;*ii*:1520.

[229] Stern J. Social mobility and the interpretation of social class mortality differentials. *J Social Policy* 1983;*12*(1):27–49.

[230] Wadsworth MEJ. Serious illness in childhood and its association with later-life achievement. In: Wilkinson RG, editor. *Class and health: research and longitudinal data*. London: Tavistock; 1986.

[231] Cochrane AL, St Leger AS and Moore F. Health Service ‘input’ and mortality ‘output’ in developed countries. *J Epidemiol Community Health* 1978;*32*:200–5.

[232] Barker DJP and Osmond C. Infant mortality, childhood nutrition, and ischemic heart disease in England and Wales. *Lancet* 1986a;*1*(8489):1077–81.

[233] Barker DJP and Osmond C. Childhood respiratory infection and adult chronic bronchitis in England and Wales. *Br Med J* 1986b;*293*:1271–5.

[234] Barker DJP and Osmond C. Inequalities in health in Britain: specific explanations in three Lancashire towns. *Br Med J* 1987;*294*:749–52.

[235] Moser KA, Fox AJ and Jones DR. Unemployment and mortality in the OPCS longitudinal study. In: Wilkinson RG, editor. *Class and health*. London: Tavistock; 1986, research and longitudinal data.

[236] Warr P. Twelve questions about unemployment and health. In: Roberts B, Finnegan R, Gallie D, editors. *New approaches to economic life*. Manchester: Manchester University Press; 1985.

[237] Desplanques G. *Mortality and activity: some aspects*. Paper to Second European Science Foundation Workshop on inequalities in health, London: City University; 1985.

[238] Part IIKawachi I and Kennedy BP. Income inequality and health: pathways and mechanisms. *Health Services Res* 1999;*34*(1):215–27.

[239] Elstad JI. The psycho-social perspective on social inequalities in health. *Sociol Health Illness* 1998;*20*(5):598–618.

[240] Nettleton S and Burrows R. Mortgage debt, insecure home ownership and health: an exploratory analysis. In: Bartley M, Blane D, Davey Smith G, editors. *The sociology of health inequalities*. Oxford: Blackwell; 1998. p. 171–92.

[241] Perry HM and Roccella EJ. Conference report on stroke mortality in the southeastern United States. *Hypertension* 1998;*31*(6):1206–15.

[242] Woodward A and Boffetta P. Environmental exposure, social class, and cancer risk. *IARC Sci Pub* 1997;*138*:361–7.

[243] Brown P. Race, class, and environmental health: a review and systematization of the literature. *Environ Res* 1995;*69*(1):15–30.

[244] Soliman MR, Derosa CT, Mielke HW and Bota K. Hazardous wastes, hazardous materials and environmental health inequity. *Toxicol Ind Health* 1993;*9*(5):901–12.

[245] Calderon RL, Johnson CC, Craun GF and Dufour AP. Health risks from contaminated water: do class and race matter? *Toxicol Ind Health* 1993;*9*(5):879–900.

[246] Sexton K, Gong Jr H, Bailar JC, Ford JG, Gold DR, Lambert WE and Utell MJ. Air pollution health risks: do class and race matter? *Toxicol Ind Health* 1993;*9*(5):843–78.

[247] Montgomery LE and Carter-Pokras O. Health status by social class and/or minority status: implications for environmental equity research. *Toxicol Ind Health* 1993;*9*(5):729–73.

[248] Suadicani P, Hein HO and Gyntelberg F. Do physical and chemical working conditions explain the association of social class with ischaemic heart disease? *Atherosclerosis* 1995;*113*(1):63–9.

[249] Boffetta P, Kogevinas M, Westerholm P and Saracci R. Exposure to occupational carcinogens and social class differences in cancer occurrence. *IARC Sci Pub* 1997;*138*:331–41.

[250] Moller H and Tonnesen H. Alcohol drinking, social class and cancer. *IARC Sci Pub* 1997;*138*:251–63.

[251] Stellman SD and Resnicow K. Tobacco smoking, cancer and social class. *IARC Sci Pub* 1997;*138*:229–50.

[252] Hemmingsson T, Lundberg I, Romelsjo A and Alfredsson L. Alcoholism in social classes and occupations in Sweden. *Int J Epidemiol* 1997;*26*(3):584–91.

[253] Blane D, Hart CL, Davey Smith G, Gillis CR, Hole DJ, Hawthorne VM. Association of cardiovascular disease risk factors with socioeconomic position during childhood and during adulthood. *Br Med J Clin Res Ed* 1996;*313*(7070):1434–8.

[254] Lowry R, Kann L, Collins JL and Kolbe LJ. The effect of socioeconomic status on chronic disease risk behaviors among US adolescents. *J Am Med Assoc* 1996; *276*(10):792–7.

[255] Blank N and Diderichsen F. Inequalities in health: the interaction between socio-economic and personal circumstances. *Public Health* 1996;*110*(3):157–62.

[256] Westin S. Mortality associated with wines, beers and spirits – study confounded by lack of correction for social class. *Br Med J* 1995;*311*(7013):1167.

[257] McGue M. The democracy of the genes. *Nature* 1997;*388*(6641):417–8.

[258] Krieger N and Sidney S. Racial discrimination and blood pressure: the CARDIA Study of young black and white adults. *Am J Public Health* 1996;*86*(10):1370–8.

[259] Brunner E. Stress and the biology of inequality. *Br Med J* 1997;*314*(7092):1472–5.

[260] Auvinen A and Karjalainen S. Possible explanations for social class differences in cancer patient survival. *IARC Sci Pub* 1997;*138*:377–97.

[261] Gergen P. Social class and asthma – distinguishing between the disease and the diagnosis. *Am J Public Health* 1996;*86*(10):1361–2.

[262] Cartwright A. Social class differences in health and care in the year before death. *J Epidemiol Community Health* 1992;*46*(1):54–7.

[263] Bartley M and Plewis I. Does health-selective mobility account for socioeconomic differences in health? Evidence from England and Wales, 1971 to 1991. *J Health Soc Behav* 1997;*38*(4):376–86.

[264] Rahkonen O, Arber S and Lahelma E. Health-related social mobility: a comparison of currently employed men and women in Britain and Finland. *Scand J Social Med* 1997;*25*(2):83–92.

[265] Stronks K, van de Mheen H, van den Bos J and Mackenbach JP. The interrelationship between income, health and employment status. *Int J Epidemiol* 1997;*26*(3):592–600.

[266] Wallace RD. Inner-city disease and the public health of the suburbs: the sociogeographic dispersion of point-source infection. *Environment Planning* 1993;*25*(12):1707–24.

[267] Rodgers B and Mann SL. Rethinking the analysis of intergenerational social mobility, social class, mental illness and social mobility – a comment on John W. Fox's "Social class, mental illness, and social mobility". *J Health Social Behav* 1993;*34*:165–72.

[268] West P. Rethinking the health selection explanation for health inequalities. *Social Sci Med* 1991;*32*:373–84.

[269] Popkin BM, Siega-Riz AM and Haines PS. A comparison of dietary trends among racial and socioeconomic groups in the United States. *New Engl J Med* 1996;*335*(10):716–20.

[270] Smith GD and Brunner E. Socio-economic differentials in health: the role of nutrition. *Proceedings of the Nutrition Society* 1997;*56*(1A):75–90.

[271] Power C and Hertzman C. Social and biological pathways linking early life and adult disease. *Br Med Bull* 1997;*53*(1):210–21.

[272] Nilsson PM, Moller L and Ostergren PO. Social class and cardiovascular disease-an update. *Scand J Social Med* 1995;*23*(1):3–8.

[273] Lasker JN, Egolf BP and Wolf S. Community social change and mortality. *Social Sci Med* 1994;*39*(1):53–62.

[274] Sclar ED. Community economic structure and individual well-being: a look behind the statistics. *Int J Health Services* 1980;*10*(4):563–79.

[275] Armstrong D, Barnett E, Casper M and Wing S. Community occupational structure, medical and economic resources, and coronary mortality among U.S. blacks and whites, 1980–1988. *Ann Epidemiol* 1998;*8*(3):184–91.

[276] Wing S, Dargent-Molina P, Casper M, Riggan W, Hayes CG, Tyroler HA. Changing association between community occupational structure and ischaemic heart disease mortality in the United States. *Lancet* 1987;*2*(8567):1067–70.

[277] Casper M, Wing S and Strogatz D. Variation in the magnitude of black-white differences in stroke mortality by community occupational structure. *J Epidemiol Community Health* 1991;*45*(4):302–6.

[278] Schoenbaum M and Waidmann T. Race, socioeconomic status and health: accounting for race differences in health. *J Gerontol* 1997;*52*(Spec No: 61–73):61–73.

[279] Lillie-Blanton M, Parsons PE, Gayle H and Dievler A. Racial differences in health: not just black and white, but shades of gray. *Annual Rev Public Health* 1996;*17*:411–48.

[280] Lillie-Blanton M and Laveist T. Race/ethnicity, the social environment, and health. *Social Sci Med* 1996;*43*(1):83–91.

[281] Bird ST. Separate black and white infant mortality models: differences in the importance of structural varables. *Social Sci Med* 1995;*41*(11):1507–12.

[282] Navarro V. Race or class or race and class: growing mortality differentials in the United States. *Int J Health Services* 1991;*21*(2):229–35.

APPENDIX TO SECTION 9

UNIT OF ANALYSIS IN A LONGITUDINAL PANEL SURVEY

In most cases, the unit of analysis in longitudinal surveys is an individual person, not the family or household. This contrasts with the usual cross-sectional surveys which, depending on their purposes, may use any one of these different units of analysis as their focus. It is very difficult to define a longitudinal family or household in any rigorous way that would enable the unit to be followed over time. New families and households are continually being created and existing ones have changing memberships. In contrast, the concept of an 'individual' is stable in a longitudinal context. Longitudinal surveys can still tell us about families and households. But the information about the families or households is derived from the individuals who are related to that particular family or household context (and their membership changes over time).

A separate but related issue concerns how one targets these individuals and their families/households: the sampling unit and the unit about which the information is to be gathered may be different. Possible sample units for a longitudinal social survey include: the individual, the household, the dwelling (or address), or the establishment. For a household panel, for instance, the target group of households in the initial wave might be gathered from either a household-based or dwelling-based sampling frame. In the latter case, the sample will be constituted by selecting the persons (and their households) within the dwelling and subsequently following them regardless of whether they continue to live in that dwelling or not.

Single indefinite life panel – individuals

In such surveys, information might be collected about the persons in a sample member's household, but no attempt is made to follow these people;

they cannot become sample members in their own right. Sometimes, however, depending on a survey's purpose, an original panel may be supplemented subsequently, e.g. by immigrants of the same birth cohort as the original sample members (OSMs). Even in this case, the focus remains on a specific class of individuals.

Single indefinite life panels – households

The rare cases where there is an attempt to use a household panel requires a more complicated design than a cohort survey because it aims to remain representative of both individuals and the households within which they reside (note that in most household panels, the population of individuals refers to the civilian non-institutional population). Mechanisms are therefore needed to ensure that there is proper representation of the populations of persons and households as time passes, in particular for representing new entrants, persons and families into that population. To ensure the on-going cross-sectional representativity of the population: 1) define all adults and children in the representative sample of households in the first wave as OSMs; and 2) in second and subsequent waves, attempt interviews with all adult members of all households containing either an OSM or an individual born to an OSM whether or not they were members of the original sample. This underlies the design of virtually all household panels. Practice differs, however, in the treatment of new panel members who subsequently stop living with an OSM.

Examples of household panel surveys include: the European Community Household Panel, the U.S. Panel Study of Income Dynamics, and the British Household Panel Survey.

Multiple overlapping fixed life panel surveys (rotating panels)

A rotating panel survey comprises a succession of separate panel surveys with staggered starting times. An initial sample of respondents is selected and interviewed a pre-determined number of times, often at intervals shorter than for most household panels. During the life of this first panel, a new sample is selected, followed, and interviewed in the same way as the first. Third and subsequent panels are constructed similarly. Thus respondents are being continuously rotated out of the survey and their numbers replenished by those being rotated into the survey. Although each constituent panel has a pre-determined fixed life, the overall survey itself usually has an indefinite life.

The rules for rotating panels are similar to those in household panels. Every adult in each household belonging to the original sample for each constituent panel is designated an OSM. All OSMs are then followed throughout the life of their panel, even if they move to a different household.

At each interview, information is collected about the OSM and the other individuals with whom they reside.

The rotating panel design has three additional features. One, the shorter interval between the interviews relative to the household panels can be used to reduce recall errors about relatively high frequency events and details of such variables as income. Second, the survey as a whole can also provide better cross-section at a point in time from the combined data from the constituent overlapping panels. The increase in sample size reduces sample errors. Third, by restricting the duration of each panel to a finite period, often only a few years, problems of attrition are reduced and representativeness more easily maintained. Examples of this approach include the U.S. Survey of Income and Program Participation (SIPP) and the Canadian Survey of Labour and Income Dynamics (SLID).

The problem with all types of longitudinal study from the point of inequalities is that sample members are lost. Whilst the nature of the longitudinal study means that one has more information on the non-responders than in a cross-sectional survey, there is still the problem that those who are lost to follow-up are likely to be different from those who remain.

INDEX